SECOND EDITION

PHYSIQUE, FITNESS, AND PERFORMANCE

SECOND EDITION

PHYSIQUE, FITNESS, AND PERFORMANCE

THOMAS BATTINELLI, Ed.D.
Professor Emeritus
Exercise and Sport Science
Fitchburg State College
Fitchburg, Massachusetts

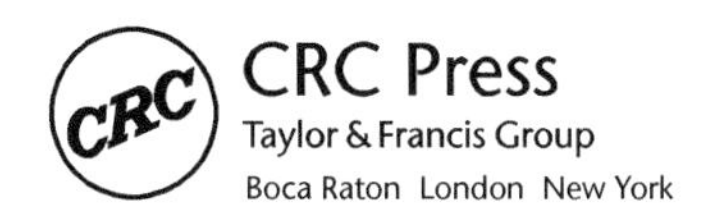

CRC Press is an imprint of the
Taylor & Francis Group, an **informa** business

CRC Press
Taylor & Francis Group
6000 Broken Sound Parkway NW, Suite 300
Boca Raton, FL 33487-2742

First issued in paperback 2019

ISBN-13: 978-0-8493-9197-2 (hbk)
ISBN-13: 978-0-367-38894-2 (pbk)

Library of Congress Cataloging-in-Publication Data

Battinelli, Thomas.
Physique, fitness, and performance / Thomas Battinelli. -- 2nd ed.
p. cm.
Includes bibliographical references and index.
ISBN 0-8493-9197-0 (alk. paper)
1. Exercise--Physiological aspects. 2. Somatotypes. 3. Physical fitness. I. Title.

QP301.B364 2007
612'.044--dc22 2007010015

Visit the Taylor & Francis Web site at
http://www.taylorandfrancis.com

and the CRC Press Web site at
http://www.crcpress.com

Dedication

To my granddaughter Sofia,
the new life in our lives

Contents

PART ONE Body Build and Body Composition

PART TWO Physical and Physiological Conditioning

PART THREE Motor Learning and Motor Control

PART FOUR Nutrition and Heart Disease

Preface

The relationship of structure to function has been substantially studied. Over the years, research results in this area of interest have well demonstrated this relationship. While physique essentially encompasses the study of body structure, body size, and body composition, fitness and performance are descriptives of the applied interaction of morphological, muscular, cardiovascular, motor, and metabolic component capacities, abilities, and skills that are developed and acquired through exercise and physical training programs.

This text has been written for undergraduate students in the exercise and sport studies who major in these fields of interest. Part One serves as the basis for the study of the structure-function relationships. Such study establishes an understanding of the history and background of the prevalent interrelationships in the study of body structure, body size, and body composition relative to fitness and physical performance. Part Two and Part Three present an overview of the quantitative and qualitative study of physical and physiological conditioning and motor learning and motor control. Quantitatively, the physical fitness health- and skill-related components are reviewed relative to training and conditioning. Qualitatively, motor ability, motor learning, and motor control are reviewed relative to the development of motor skill within general and specific parameter guidelines. Fatigue, the inevitable result of exercise and performance, provides a further analysis of the physiological and psychological training processes. Part Four provides the fundamental understandings to the physiological processes that occur during exercise relative to nutrient function. This section also presents coverage on the relationships of nutrition and obesity to heart disease. Part Five, the appendix section, includes the pertinent figures, tables, and forms used in evaluation and programming.

Thomas Battinelli

Acknowledgments

The author wishes to acknowledge the assistance of the following individuals in the preparation and completion of this textbook: Robert A. Foley, M.L.S., Director of Library, Fitchburg State College; Jeremiah E. Greene, M.L.S., librarian, Fitchburg State College; Bruce Mc Sheehy, M.A., librarian, Fitchburg State College; Jean W. Missud, M.A., librarian, Fitchburg State College; Mary E. Leger, Inter Library Loan Services, Fitchburg State College; Paulette M. Rameau, secretary, Fitchburg State College; Regina M. Pisa, J.D., managing partner, Goodwin Procter Law Firm; Stephen Charkoudian, J.D., partner, Goodwin Proctor Law Firm, Zheng-Yi Chen, Ph.D., assistant professor of neuroscience/researcher, Harvard Medical School and Massachusetts General Hospital; Elisabeth M. Battinelli, M.D., Ph. D., hematology-oncology clinical fellow, Beth Israel Deaconess Medical Center.

The Author

Thomas Battinelli is a professor emeritus from the Exercise and Sport Science Department at Fitchburg State College in Fitchburg, Massachusetts. He received his Bachelor of Science degree in physical education from Boston University, his Master of Education degree in educational administration from Boston College, and his Doctoral Degree in health and human movement from Boston University. Dr. Battinelli has presented research papers regionally, nationally, and internationally, authored numerous research studies and articles, and has had two books published. His research areas range from studies on body build and physical performance, to motor ability and motor learning, philosophy and physical education, exercise and nutrition, and administration and athletics. These studies were published in *The Journal of Human Biology, The British Journal of Sports Medicine, The International Journal of Physical Education, The Journal of Teaching in Physical Education, The Physical Educator, Athletic Administration, Rivista di Cultura Sportiva,* and *Annali.* He also collaborated as a principal investigator for Fitchburg State College with University of Massachusetts Epidemiological Researchers in studies on Cholesterol and Calcium.

During his tenure at Fitchburg State College, Dr. Battinelli was a faculty member for 47 years, athletic director for 10 years, and department chair for 30 years. He has been both college active and community active. In reference to college activities, he was chair of the Athletic Council and served as a member of the Academic Policies, the Department Chairs, the Institutional Wellness, and the Human Studies Committees. As for his community activities, Dr. Battinelli has been involved in public school physical education advisory work, served as governor on the Administrative Board of the Dante Alighieri Cultural Society, and currently is an operations volunteer for the Somerville Museum. In regard to honors and awards, Dr. Battinelli has been a recipient of an Honor Award from the Massachusetts Association for Health, Physical Education, Recreation, and Dance, received two Distinguished Service Awards, and won the Mara Award for Teaching Excellence from Fitchburg State College.

Part One

Body Build and Body Composition

1 Physique, Fitness, and Performance

INTRODUCTION

The relationship of physique to fitness and performance has been substantially studied. Over the years, research results in this area of interest have well demonstrated this relationship well. While physique essentially encompasses the study of body structure, body size, and body composition, fitness and performance are descriptive of the applied interaction of morphological, muscular, cardiovascular, motor, and metabolic component capacities, abilities, and skills that are developed and acquired through exercise and physical training programs.[2,3]

BODY BUILD AND BODY COMPOSITION: THE PHYSIQUE COMPONENTS

Physique or body build can be characterized by the interactive sum of its parts, body structure, body size, and body composition. (Figure 1.1).[1,2,3,9]

1. Body structure — the distributive component parts of the body
2. Body size — the body mass, volume, length, and surface area of the body
3. Body composition — the fat and fat-free ratio percentage components of the body

In relation to measurement and assessment, three major interrelated but somewhat dichotomous classification systems of study have emerged through the years (Table 1.1). The physique rating systems include those of body type, somatotype, and anthropometric somatotype. These classification forms of study have focused on the measure of structure, shape, and form through anthroposcopic and anthropometric methods of evaluation. The body build index rating systems include those of factor type, body type, dysplasia type, and proportionality assessments. These rating systems are index oriented and utilize anthropometric length, breadth, and circumference methods of assessment to identify and relate body measures to one another in the form of ratios. Through the use of statistical computations, body build assessments and classifications have been made relative to size, proportionality, and disproportionality. The last, but probably the most recently utilized systems of study, have been those in the field of body composition. Laboratory and field methods of

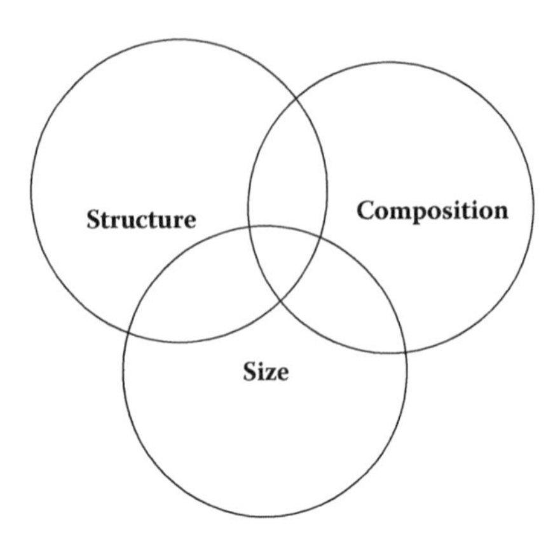

FIGURE 1.1 Physique components. (From Bioleau, R.A. and T.H. Lohman, *Orthopedic Clinics of North America,* 8, 563–581, 1977. With the permission of the publisher.)

TABLE 1.1
Body Build and Body Composition: The Physique Components

The Physique Components

Body Build	Body Build Indices	Body Composition
Body Types	Factor Types	Densitometric
Somatotypes	Dysplasia Types	Dilutional
Anthropometric	Body Size	Nitrogen
Somatotypes		Potassium
		X-Ray
		Ultrasound
		Anthropometric
		Computed Tomography
		Magnetic Resonance
		Electrical Conductivity Infrared Interactance
		Photon Absorptiometry
		Air Displacement Plethysmography

assessment have generally incorporated densitometric, dilutional, nitrogen, potassium, x-ray, ultrasound, anthropometric, computed tomography, magnetic resonance, electrical conductivity, infrared interactance, photon absorptiometry, and air displacement plethysmography evaluations to measure fat and fat-free body weight.

To date, research in these areas of study have demonstrated the morphological, biomechanical, and physiological influence of structure, size, and composition on performance.[1,5,7,8,13–22] A summary of these findings generally indicate that:

1. The position of muscular attachments, the structural size of joints, and the length of bones can either enhance or limit function.
2. Body build can set influential limits for performance but does not control the capacity for work.
3. Proportionality in size and shape can constitute specific prerequisites for successful performance.
4. Muscle force is directly related to muscle cross section.
5. Structure–function interactions can be interpreted through length, mass, and time studies, and their derivatives can be expressed in physiological terms.
6. Environmental, biomechanical, and morphological constraints on performance can include the factors of spatial and temporal controls, physical laws and principles, and overall size and form measures.
7. The amount of fat-free and fat weight can be of positive and/or negative value in regard to performance.
8. Generally, mesomorphs have been found to be stronger and more agile, and to possess more muscular endurance than ectomorphs and endomorphs.

CONDITIONING AND TRAINING: THE PHYSICAL FITNESS COMPONENTS

Physical fitness can be defined as the capacity to do physical work within gradated levels of performance quantitatively and qualitatively (Table 1.2). The quantitative training parameters are health related and include the components of muscular strength, muscular endurance, flexibility, and cardiovascular endurance:

1. Muscular strength — the maximal repetitive or sustained exertion of force against resistance
2. Muscular endurance — the submaximal repetitive or sustained exertion of force against resistance
3. Flexibility — the functional joint movement of the body and limbs through a range of movement
4. Cardiovascular endurance — the contributive metabolic energy force that is descriptive of the physiological work capacity of the body relative to the performance efficiency of the vascular and respiratory heart and lungs over extended periods of time

TABLE 1.2
Physical Fitness: The Conditioning and Training Components

Physical Fitness:

The Conditioning and Training Components

Health Related	**Skill Related**
Muscular Strength	**Agility**
Muscular Endurance	**Balance**
Flexibility	**Coordination**
Cardiovascular	**Speed**
Endurance	**Power**

The qualitative training parameters are skill related in nature and include the components of agility, balance, coordination, speed, and power.

1. Agility — the ability to change direction quickly and accurately while in movement
2. Balance — vestibular function and the state of equilibrium during static and dynamic activity
3. Coordination — the learned execution of movement patterns
4. Speed — the repetitive movement of body limbs related to the coverage of distance or periods of time as quickly as possible
5. Power — the amount of explosive force exerted as quickly as possible over a designated bodily range distance

GENERAL MOTOR ABILITY AND SPECIFIC MOTOR ABILITY: THE MOTOR COMPONENTS

Ability or general motor ability can be defined as the inherited and learned capacity demonstrated in the performance of fundamental skill activities.[11] Components such as muscular strength, muscular endurance, power, speed, cardiovascular endurance, flexibility, agility, and coordination were established, and tests were developed as measures of these factors (Table 1.3). Measures of this type were aimed at the predictive evaluation of physical performance and the generality and the transferability of skill activities.[4,5] Later studies in this field of research, however, disputed such general findings. Subsequent investigations were more demonstrative of the specificities in movement parameters (Table 1.3). The later theories were more motor skill and neuromotor centered and considered to be independent and nontransferable

TABLE 1.3
General and Specific Motor Ability: The Motor Components

General and Specific Motor Ability:
The Motor Components
General Motor Ability
Muscular Strength
Muscular Endurance
Power
Speed
Cardiovascular Endurance
Flexibility
Agility
Coordination
Specific Motor Ability
Specific Motor Skills Related to Designated Physical Activity Movement Parameters.

relative to the performance specificities derived from undertaken physical tasks.[9] Subsequent studies in the generality–specificity controversy were demonstrative of an ability to skill construct.[6] This construct model was indicative of the practice and learning changes that were inherent in the training process. Motor abilities formed the basic general abilities of the initial stages of learning that became more motor-skill specific with practice in the later stages of learning. In addition, motor learning and motor control are the interconnected areas of study that provide the coordinative processes and mechanisms underlying the learning and acquiring of motor skills.

NUTRIENT AND ENERGY UTILIZATION: THE METABOLIC COMPONENTS

Nutrition can be defined as the intake, transformation, and utilization of food substances. In relation to physical activity, nutrition provides the fundamental understandings to the physiological processes that occur during exercise relative to nutrient function. The basic nutrients, carbohydrates, fats, proteins, vitamins, minerals, and water, are functionally used by the body for energy metabolism during physical work. Metabolically, the development of aerobic and anaerobic conditioning through physical training is significant to overall cardiovascular fitness and function (Table 1.4). Aerobic endurance is gained through work in the presence of oxygen, while anaerobic conditioning is attained through work without the presence of oxygen. Both of these systems work in conjunction with one another, utilizing appropriate aerobic and anaerobic metabolic processes to a greater and/or lesser extent depending on bodily needs in response to exercise. The nutrient and energy responses produced by these systems contribute to the resulting physiological work capacity of the body in regard to physical performance.

TABLE 1.4
Energy Systems and Energy Sources Utilization: The Metabolic Components

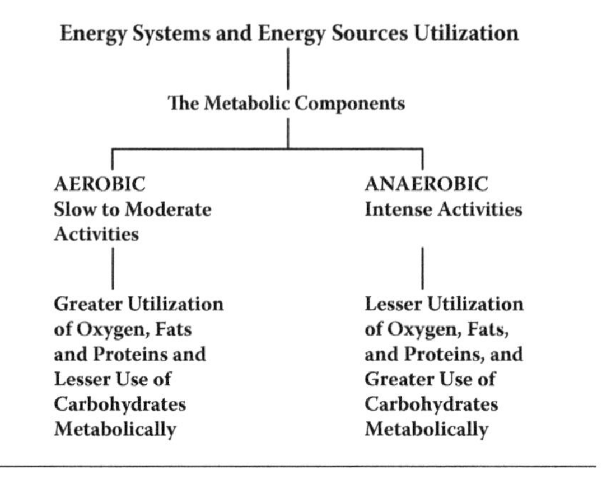

PHYSICAL PERFORMANCE

Physical performance can be described as the increased synergistic patterning of proficiency and competency acquired through the conditioning and training of developed structural and functional capacities, abilities, and skills relative to nutrient and metabolic utilization that can be demonstrated during the execution of designated physical activities (Table 1.5). Physiological and psychological fatigue must also be considered in this process as a resultant effect factor relative to work decrement. In

TABLE 1.5
Physical Performance

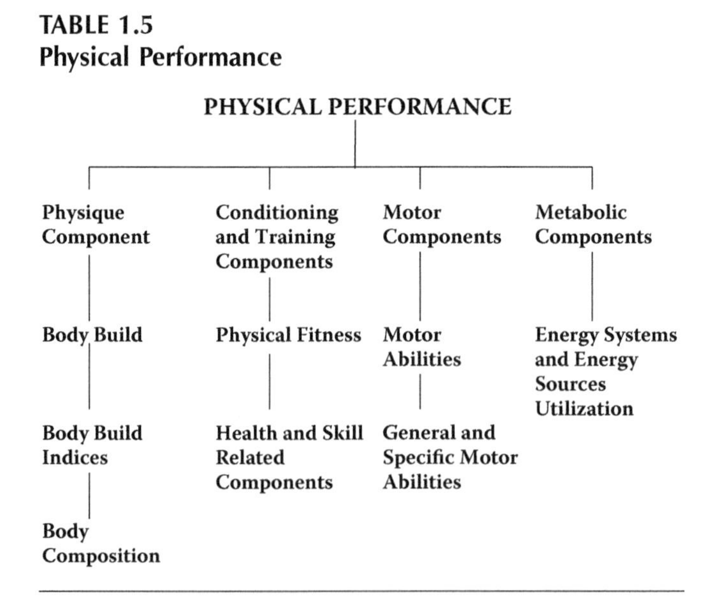

essence, physical performance can be the capstone of these integrative systems that must work together in the pursuit of the movement goals sought. These goals are quantitative and qualitative in nature and form the basis for the structure–function relationships that are indigenous to physique, fitness, and physical performance.

PHYSIQUE, EXERCISE, NUTRITION, AND HEART DISEASE

The relationship of physique, exercise, and nutrition to heart disease must also be considered. Studies have shown that physique, namely the endomorphic and mesomorphic body builds, can be significantly related to high cholesterol levels and the subsequent higher risks of heart disease.[5] Exercise in this relationship has been generally efficacious and has been shown to lower total cholesterol, low-density lipoprotein, and triglycerides, and to increase high-density lipoprotein.[10] Nutrition has also played a role in this relationship, since healthful and nutritional diets have also been reported to lower cholesterol levels. The subsequent effects of exercise and diet on physique, blood lipids, and lipoproteins can therefore be beneficial toward the promotion of overall health and fitness.

SUMMARY

The relationship of physique to fitness and performance has been substantially studied. Over the years, results in this area of interest have well demonstrated this relationship. A summary of the findings have generally indicated that:

1. Physique or body build can be characterized by the interactive sum of its parts, body structure, body size, and body composition.
2. Physical fitness can be defined as the capacity to do physical work within gradated levels of performance quantitatively and qualitatively.
3. The quantitative parameters are health related and include the components of muscular strength, muscular endurance, flexibility, and cardiovascular endurance.
4. The qualitative parameters are skill related and include the components of agility, balance, coordination, speed, and power.
5. Ability or general motor ability can be defined as the inherited and learned capacity demonstrated in the performance of fundamental skill activities.
6. Later theories were more motor skill and neuromotor centered and considered to be independent and nontransferable relative to the performance specificities derived from undertaken physical tasks.
7. In relation to physical activity, nutrition provides the fundamental understanding to the physiological processes that occur during exercise relative to nutrient function.
8. The basic nutrients, carbohydrates, fats, proteins, vitamins, minerals, and water, are functionally used by the body for energy metabolism during physical work.

9. Physical performance can be described as the increased synergistic patterning of proficiency and competency acquired through the conditioning and training of developed structural and functional capacities, abilities, and skills relative to nutrient and metabolic utilization that can be demonstrated during the execution of designated physical activities.
10. Studies have shown that physique, namely the endomorphic and mesomorphic body builds, can be significantly related to high cholesterol levels and subsequent higher risks of heart disease.

GLOSSARY

Aerobic Physical work done in the presence of oxygen
Agility Rapid change of direction while in movement
Air displacement plethysmography The measure of the air displacement volume of the body to determine the body composition values of fat and fat-free ratios
Anaerobic Physical work done without the presence of oxygen
Anthropometric somatotype Physique rating component system of live body measurement classification
Anthropometry Quantitative measures of selected human landmarks
Anthroposcopy Visual study of bodily features and form
Balance Body equilibrium
Biomechanics The science of body movement
Body composition The fat and fat-free tissues of the body
Body proportionality/disproportionality Common and/or variational similarities and/or differences, respectively, in body size and body shape
Body size The physical height and mass or weight of the body
Body structure The basic build of the body
Body type Physique rating type system of classification
Carbohydrates Compounds that contain carbon, hydrogen, and oxygen atoms in polysaccharide, disaccharide, and monosaccharide formations
Cardiovascular endurance The stamina that can be demonstrated during prolonged physical activity
Cholesterol A sterol, an essential metabolite, and a fatlike substance
Computed tomography The use of x-ray beam scanning procedures to produce a cross-sectional image of the fat and fat-free tissues of the body
Coordination Learned movement pattern that is the resultant of the integrated unity of singular skills
Densitometric (underwater weighing) The measure of specific gravity and body density through water volume displacement of weight in air and weight in water
Dilutional (total body water) The use of isotopic deuterium and tritium oxide dilutions to estimate water content and body cellular mass
Dysplasia/disproportions Variational body regional differences in physique rating relative to given norm ranges

Ectomorphy Somatotype predominance of linearity and fragility

Electrical conductivity (total body) Electromagnetic radiation waves used to measure the electrolyte tissue content and electrical conductivity flow through the body

Endomorphy Somatotype predominance of roundness and softness

Factor types The body build variability or types that have been identified and quantified

Fat body weight The fat component of body weight

Fats Compounds that contain carbon, hydrogen, and oxygen and are classified as triglycerides, phospholipids, and cholesterol

Flexibility The extent to which a muscle or group of muscles can functionally move through a range of motion around a joint

Frame size The basic build of the body determined by the proportional relationship of height to one or more breadth measures

General motor ability The general underlying capacity of an individual to perform a number of physical skills

High-density lipoproteins Lipoproteins that are small in size, dense in weight, and are the main carriers of cholesterol from body tissues

Infrared interactance The use of an electromagnetic radiation body probe to measure the absorptive and reflective spectrographic chemical properties of fat, water, and protein

Lean body weight The fat-free component of body weight

Low-density lipoproteins Lipoproteins that contain mostly cholesterol and are the prime carriers of this sterol to body tissues

Magnetic resonance The use of magnetic scanning procedures to produce a cross-sectional image of the fat and fat-free tissues of the body

Mesomorphy Somatotype predominance of squareness and hardness

Minerals Inorganic substances that act as regulatory agents in the body

Morphology The study of human form and structure

Muscular endurance Submaximal repetitive or sustained muscular exertion force against a resistance

Muscular strength Maximal exertion of force against resistance during one trial effort

Nitrogen (total body) The measurement of total body nitrogen through gamma ray immersions used to determine the amount of protein in muscle and nonmuscle tissue

Photon absorptiometry (dual body) Two-energy-level photon scans of the body through which the energy differences observed can determine the mineral bone mass of the body

Physical fitness The capacity to do physical work within gradated levels of performance quantitatively and qualitatively

Physique/body build Body structure, body size, and body composition

Potassium (total body) The gamma ray measure of the potassium content of the body used to determine the cellular mass of muscle and nonmuscle components

Power The amount of work performed per unit of time

Proteins Compounds that contain carbon, hydrogen, and oxygen and are constructed of linked chains of amino acids
Somatotype Physique rating component system of classification
Specific motor ability Abilities that are specific to the nature of the skill to be performed
Speed Rapidity in repeated patterns of movement
Triglycerides Fat compounds that contain glycerol and three fatty acids
Ultrasound The use of high-frequency sound waves to identify and quantify the density levels of body tissues
Vitamins Organic compounds that act as biochemical catalysts in the transformation of food into energy
X-ray Radiographic analysis of the thickness levels of bone, muscle, and fat

REFERENCES

1. Abernathy, B. et al., *The Biophysical Foundations of Human Movement,* 2nd ed., Human Kinetics Publishers, Champaign, IL, 2005.
2. Bloomfield, J., T.R. Ackland, and B.C. Elliott, *Applied Anatomy and Biomechanics in Sport*, Blackwell Scientific Publications, Boston, 1994.
3. Bioleau, R.A. and T.H. Lohman, The measurement of human physique and its effects on physical performance, *Orthopedic Clinics of North America,* 8, 563–581, 1977.
4. Bouchard, C., R.J. Shephard, and T. Stephens, Eds., *Physical Activity, Fitness, and Health Consensus Statement,* Human Kinetics Publishers, Champaign, IL, 1993.
5. Carter, J.E.L. and B.H. Heath, *Somatotyping — Development and Applications*, Cambridge University Press, Cambridge, 1990.
6. Fleishman, E.A., On the relation between abilities, learning, and human performance, *American Psychologist,* 27, 1017–1032, 1972.
7. Heath, B.H. and J.E.L. Carter, A modified somatotype method, *American Journal of Physical Anthropology*, 27, 57–74, 1967.
8. Higgins, J.R., *Human Movement: An Integrated Approach*, C.V. Mosby Company, St. Louis, 1977.
9. Houthkouper, L.B. and S.B. Goring, Body composition: How should it be measured? Does it affect sport performance? *Sport Science Exchange*, 7, 1–10, 1994.
10. Kwiterovich, P.O., *The Johns Hopkins Complete Guide for Preventing and Reversing Heart Disease,* Prima Publishing, Rocklin, CA, 1993.
11. Magill, R.A., *Motor Learning and Control: Concepts and Applications*, 7th ed., McGraw-Hill, Dubuque, IA, 2004.
12. Schmidt, R.A. and T. D. Lee, *Motor Control and Learning, A Behavioral Emphasis,* 3rd ed., Human Kinetics Publishers, Champaign, IL, 2005.
13. Schmidt, R.A., *Motor Learning and Performance,* 3rd ed., Human Kinetics Publishers, Champaign, IL, 2004.
14. Sheldon, W.H., S.S. Stevens, and W.B. Tucker, *The Varieties of Human Physique,* Harper and Brothers, New York, 1940.
15. Shepard, R.J., Physical activity, fitness, and health: the current consensus, *Quest*, 47, 288–303, 1995.
16. Sills, F.D. and P.W. Everett, The relationship of extreme somatotypes to performance in motor and strength tests, *Research Quarterly*, 24, 223–228, 1953.

17. Simon, E., *Morphological Development and Functional Efficiency: International Research in Sport and Physical Education,* Charles C Thomas, Springfield, IL, 1964.
18. Tanner, J.M., Growth and constitution, in *Anthropology Today,* Kroeber, A.L., Ed., The University of Chicago Press, Chicago, 1954.
19. Tanner, J.M., *The Physique of the Olympic Athlete,* Allen and Unwin, London, 1964.
20. Whitney, E. and S.R. Rolfes, *Understanding Nutrition,* 10th ed., Thomson Wadsworth, Belmont, CA, 2005.
21. Wilmore, J.H., Design issues and alternatives in assessing physical fitness among apparently healthy adults in a health examination survey of the general population, in *Assessing Physical Fitness and Physical Activity in Population Based Surveys,* National Center for Health Statistics, Washington, DC, 1990.
22. Wilmore, J.H., *Physiology of Sport and Exercise,* 3rd ed., Human Kinetics Publishers, Champaign, IL: 2004.

2 Body Build and Body Build Indices

INTRODUCTION

The relationship of body build or physique to physical performance and activity has been substantially investigated within given fields of interest. Over the years, the structure, size, and function relationships have been well established and generally accepted by researchers and practitioners in these fields. Research in this area of study has been centered on the development of morphological rating systems of assessment and classification and the application of these systems to physical performance (Figure 2.1).

BODY TYPES

Human morphological measurement can be traced back to the physique classification established by Hippocrates[2,74] He designated two main physical types: the phthisic habitus (tall and thin) and the apoplectic habitus (short and thick). After the inception of this two-pole system, subsequent formulations also designated disparate types and established distinct extreme categories, within which intermediate physical types were sometimes classified. Such evaluations were subjective in nature and based on the anthroposcopic (visual) study of bodily features and form. The physique types established by Hippocrates remained as a standard measure of the human form, and few advances were made until 1797, when Gall and Spurzheim developed a three-pole system that included the type digestif (digestive), type musculaire (muscular), and type cerebral (cerebral).[78]

The advent of the science of anthropometry (quantitative measures of selected human body landmarks) furthered the cause of human morphological measurement. In 1909 Viola became the first anthropologist to present a comprehensive system for the external measurement of the body.[72] His formulations were based on ten measures of trunk volume and extremity lengths, compared to established norm values, and placed on a linearity/nonlinearity scale continuum. His physique classification included the following types: macrosplanchnic (large heavy trunk and short limbs), normosplanchnic (medium trunk and medium limbs), and microsplanchnic (small trunk and long limbs). The next noted classification system based on pole types was devised by Kretschmer.[20,44,63,67] He became the first psychologist to relate morphological body build to mental characteristics. His three types, similar to those proposed earlier by others, were different in that they were more representative of

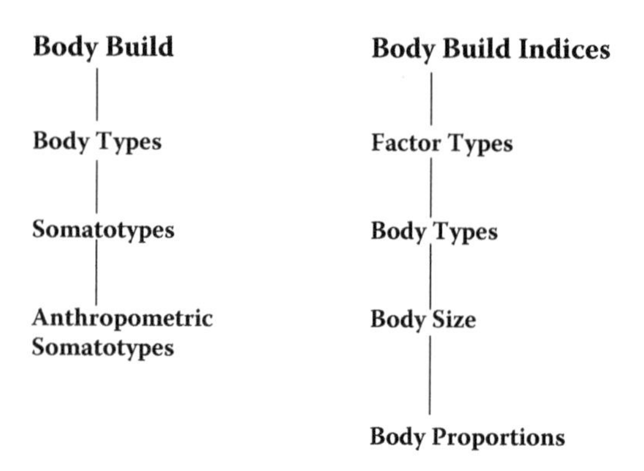

FIGURE 2.1 Body build and body build indices.

extreme combinations of variables within an established continuum. His classification system included the following types: pyknic (corpulent), athletic (stocky), and asthenic (slender).

SOMATOTYPES

Probably the most advanced classification system of the mid-twentieth century was that proposed by Sheldon.[4,5,10,11,28,63] Having been influenced by the works of Viola and Kretschmer, he developed a somatotype rating system that was based on component variables instead of types. His somatotype was derived from the endodermal, mesodermal, and ectodermal embryonic tissue layers and formed what he termed the endomorphic (roundness and softness), mesomorphic (squareness and hardness), and ectomorphic (linearity and fragility) components of body build. These component variables were quantitative in nature, in that equal minimal to maximal interval levels were established to provide a diverse, but yet to some degree continuous, system. Photographs were taken and, through utilization of both anthroposcopic and anthropometric methods of measurement, scaled to size (Figure 2.2).[76] Endomorphic, mesomorphic, and ectomorphic evaluations were derived from measures of the head and neck, upper and lower trunks, and arm and leg body landmark regions.

ANTHROPOMETRIC SOMATOTYPES

Further advances in morphological rating systems were made by Parnell.[55] While his physique rating component classification was similar to that established by Sheldon, Parnell utilized live body measurements (skinfold, bone, circumference, height, and weight) to obtain what was termed an anthropometric somatotype. His component designations were fat, muscularity, and linearity, set within interval ranges of one through seven. A physique deviation chart was used to enter the selected measurements, and processes were established to obtain an objective rating of body build.

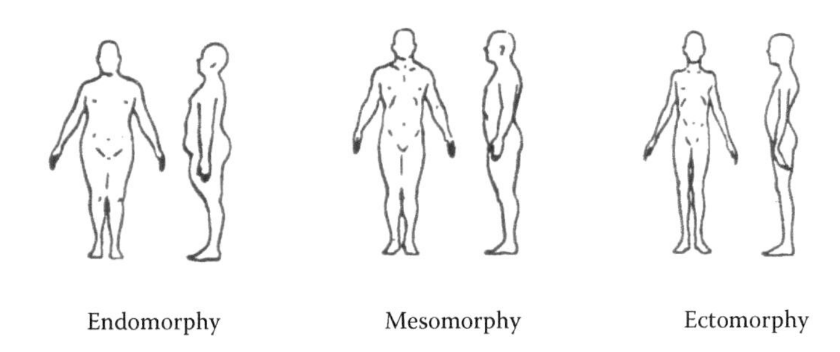

FIGURE 2.2 Extreme somatotypes. (From Van Huss, et al., *Physical Activity in Modern Living*, 2nd ed., Prentice-Hall, Englewood Cliffs, NJ, 1969. Allyn and Bacon, 1969. Reprinted by permission of Pearson Education.)

Although a number of somatotype modification systems have been developed in recent years, the most prominent, practical, and utilized anthropometric somatotype classification has probably been that established by Heath and Carter.[10,11,18,33,34] Similar in component designations endomorphy, mesomorphy, and ectomorphy to those incorporated by Sheldon, and similar to the live-body measurement processes developed by Parnell, the Heath–Carter system was nevertheless different in that it presented a descriptive somatotype rating not related to genetic tendencies relative to age and not restricted to established interval ranges. Quantitative skinfold, breadth, circumference, height, and weight measures are taken and then entered on a somatotype rating form (Appendix 1).[18] Assessment procedures were calculative in process with endomorphic fatness, mesomorphic muscularity, and ectomorphic body size levels incorporated into an anthropometric somatogram description of the somatotype ratings obtained (Figure 2.3).[18]

Further advances in somatotype anthropometry will probably be related to methodological development. The use of computerized axial tomography and magnetic resonance imaging will provide additional information relative to the internal masses of the body.[11,19] The incorporation of this data into that of present systems in use today will enhance the quantifiable assessment of the structure, size, and composition of the body.[13]

BODY BUILD AND PHYSICAL PERFORMANCE

Somatotype and anthropometric somatotype assessments in the study of physical performance have been designed to measure the general and/or specific physique, size, shape, and form indigenous to the athletes and the activities being studied. In the past, research-oriented assessments were subjective in nature, with photometric techniques utilized relative to body-build evaluations projected from picture form to live body representations.[73] Recent research developments, however, have enabled investigators to use live body anthropometric measures of assessment.[35]

Studies on the somatotypes of athletes, elite athletes, and Olympic athletes have generally shown that (Tables 2.1, 2.2 and 2.3):[3,4,5,10,11,17,22–24,35,38,49,52,53,56–58,65,66,70,73,80–84]

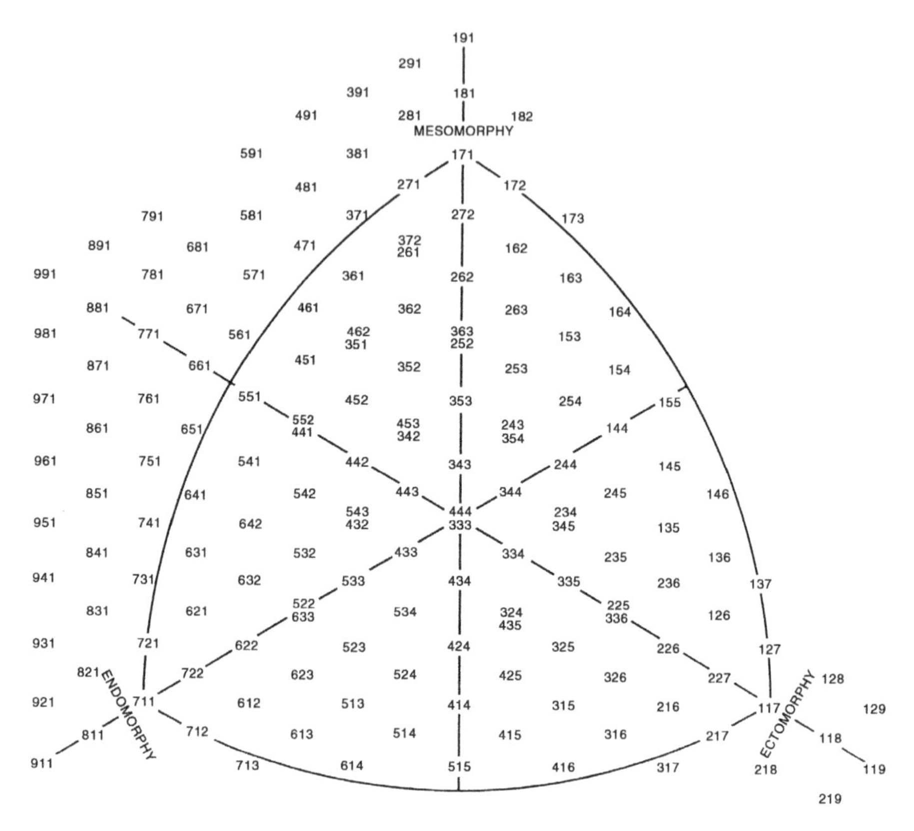

FIGURE 2.3 Somatochart. (From Carter, J.E.L., and B.H. Heath, *Somatotyping-Development Applications,* Cambridge University Press, Cambridge, 1990. Reprinted with the permission of Cambridge University Press.)

1. Strength- and speed-dependent athletes tended to be basically mesomorphic.
2. Distance-dependent athletes were found to be more ectomorphic, with limited amounts of mesomorphic muscularity.
3. Male athletes were more mesomorphic, but less endomorphic and ectomorphic, than their female counterparts.
4. In reference to the male athletes, weight lifters were more endomorphic and mesomorphic, but less ectomorphic, than were the boxers and judo competitors. Gymnasts and canoeists were more mesomorphic and less endomorphic than were the fencers, field hockey players, cyclists, and rowers.
5 In reference to the somatotypes of female athletes, gymnasts and track and field athletes were less endomorphic than were the canoeists, rowers, and swimmers.
6. Decathlon and pentathlon athletes were more mesomorphic and less ectomorphic than were the jumpers and throwers.
7. Mesomorphs were found to be superior to their endomorphic and ectomorphic counterparts in terms of strength, speed, and agility.

TABLE 2.1
Somatotypes of Male Athletes

Athletic Group or Sport	n	Age (yrs)	Height (cm)	Weight (kg)	Somatotype Endo	Somatotype Meso	Somatotype Ecto	Reference
Runners:								
Sprint	78	23.9	175.4	68.4	1.7	5.0	2.8	de Garay et al.
Middle Distance	41	22.9	177.3	65.0	1.5	4.2	3.6	
Long Distance	34	25.3	171.9	59.8	1.4	4.1	3.6	
	19	—	174.4	60.8	2.7	4.2	4.3	Tanner
Marathon	20	26.4	168.7	56.6	1.4	4.3	3.5	de Garay et al.
	9	—	171.1	59.9	2.6	4.4	3.9	Tanner
Track and Field:								
Jumpers	31	23.5	182.8	73.2	1.7	4.4	3.4	de Garay et al.
Weight throwers	14	27.3	186.1	102.3	3.5	7.1	1.0	
Weight Lifters	59	26.7	168.0	76.6	2.4	7.1	1.0	
Wrestlers	49	25.8	169.3	70.6	2.2	6.3	1.6	
	32	—	172.4	72.0	2.7	5.6	2.5	Tanner
Swimmers	65	19.2	179.3	72.1	2.1	5.0	2.9	de Garay et al.

Source: From Wilmore, J.H., C.H. Brown, and J.A. Davis, *Annals of the New York Academy of Science*, 301, 764–776, 1977. Permission granted by the Annals of the New York Academy of Sciences.

TABLE 2.2
Somatotypes of Female Athletes

Athletic Group or Sport	n	Age (yrs)	Height (cm)	Weight (kg)	Somatotype Endo	Somatotype Meso	Somatotype Ecto	Reference
Runners:								
Sprint	28	20.7	16.0	56.8	2.7	3.9	2.9	de Garay et al.
Middle Distance	18	20.0	166.9	54.3	2.0	3.3	3.7	
Track and Field:								
Jumpers	12	21.5	169.4	56.4	2.2	3.3	3.7	de Garay et al.
Weight throwers	9	19.9	170.9	73.5	5.3	5.2	1.7	
Swimmers	28	16.3	164.4	56.9	3.4	4.0	3.0	de Garay et al.

Source: From Wilmore, J.H., C.H. Brown, and J.A. Davis, *Annals of the New York Academy of Science*, 301, 764–776, 1977. Permission granted by the Annals of the New York Academy of Sciences.

8. The somatotypes of athletes within given sports activities, although similar, were dissimilar relative to size and proportions within given events and positional play.
9. The somatotypes of champion athletes were progressively more similar relative to size and proportions as competitive levels increased in regard to given sports activities and to given events and positional play.

TABLE 2.3
Somatotypes of High-Level Sportsmen and Sportswomen

Sport	Males	Females
Racquet sports		
Tennis	2.0–4.5–3.0	3.5–3.5–3.0
Badminton	2.5–4.5–3.0	— — —
Squash	2.5–5.0–3.0	3.5–4.0–3.0
Racquetball	3.0–3.5–3.0	— — —
Aquatic sports		
Swimming	2.0–5.0–3.0	3.0–4.0–3.0
Waterpolo	2.5–5.5–2.5	3.5–4.0–3.0
Rowing	2.5–5.5–2.5	3.0–4.0–3.0
Canoeing	2.0–5.5–2.5	3.0–4.5–2.5
Gymnastic and power sports		
Gymnastics	1.5–6.0–2.0	2.0–4.0–3.0
		*
Skating	1.5–5.0–3.0	2.5–4.0–3.0
Diving	2.0–5.5–2.5	3.0–4.0–3.0
Weightlifting (<60 kg)	1.5–7.0–1.0	— — —
(60–79.9 kg)	2.0–7.0–1.0	— — —
(80–99.9 kg)	2.5–8.0–0.5	— — —
(>100 kg)	5.0–9.0–0.5	— — —
Track, field and cycling		
Sprint running and hurdles	1.5–5.0–3.0†	2.5–4.0–3.0
400 m, 400 m hurdles	1.5–4.5–3.5	2.0–3.5–3.5
800 m, 1500 m	1.5–4.5–3.5	2.0–3.5–3.5
5000 m, 10,000 m	1.5–4.0–3.5	— — —
Marathon	1.5–4.5–3.5	
Shot, discus, hammer	3.0–7.0–1.0	5.5–5.5–1.5
High, long, triple jump	1.5–4.0–3.5	2.5–3.0–4.0
Cycling: Track	2.0–5.5–2.5	— — —
Road	1.5–4.5–3.0	— — —
Mobile field sports		
Field hockey	2.5–4.5–2.5	— — —
Soccer	2.5–5.0–2.5	4.0–4.5–2.0
Lacrosse	3.0–5.5–2.5	4.0–4.5–2.5
Contact field sports		
Rugby	3.0–6.0–2.0	— — —
Australian football	2.0–5.5–2.5	— — —
American football: Linemen	5.0–7.5–1.0	— — —
Backs	3.0–5.5–1.5	— — —
Set field sports		
Baseball (males only), softball (females only)	2.5–5.5–2.0	3.5–4.5–2.0

TABLE 2.3 ***(Continued)***
Somatotypes of High-Level Sportsmen and Sportswomen

Sport		Males	Females
Cricket		— — —	5.0–4.5–2.0
Golf		4.0–5.0–2.0	4.0–4.0–2.5
Court sports			
Basketball		2.0–4.5–3.5	4.0–4.0–3.0
Netball		— — —	3.0–4.0–3.5
Volleyball		2.5–4.5–3.5	3.5–4.0–3.0
Martial arts			
Judo		2.0–6.5–1.5	4.0–4.0–2.0
Wrestling	(<60 kg)	1.5–5.5–2.5	— — —
	(60–79.9 kg)	2.0–6.5–1.5	— — —
	(80–99.9 kg)	2.5–7.0–1.0	— — —
	(>100 kg)	4.0–7.5–1.0	— — —
Boxing	(<60 kg)	1.5–5.0–3.0	— — —
	(60–79.9 kg)	2.0–5.5–2.5	— — —
	(80–89.9 kg)	2.5–6.0–2.0	— — —

* More mature gymnastis 3.0–4.0–3.0.
† Most specialist 100 m sprinters score at least 5.5 on mesomorphy.

Source: From Bloomfield, J., T.R. Ackland, and B.C. Elliott, *Applied Anatomy and Biomechanics in Sport,* Blackwell Scientific Publications, Boston, 1994. Permission granted by Blackwell Science Asia P/L.

In regard to athlete variability in size and proportional build within given sports activities, Leake and Carter[45] found female triathletes to be generally heavier, more mesomorphic, and less ectomorphic than elite runners. Foley et al.[27] also found that cyclists differed structurally relative to their event specializations. Sprinters were more mesomorphic and shorter, while time tourists were more ectomorphic and taller. These results were corroborated by Orvanova[54] in her study on weight lifters. She found that, while those in the lighter weight classes were classified as ectomorphic or balanced mesomorphs, those in the heavier weight classes were found to be endomorphic mesomorphs. In reference to elite volleyball players, Gualdi-Russo and Zaccagni[30] reported that the physique of these athletes was high in ectomorphy and low in endomorphy and mesomorphy.

Somatotype adaptations due to physical training and competitive participation over the seasonal course of play have also been studied. Carter and Phillips[21] reported an endomorphic decrease for males in an exercise program over a two-year period. Carter and Rahe,[20] in a four-month study on underwater demolition training participants, found decreases in all three endomorphic, mesomorphic, and ectomorphic components during that period of time. A similar study on football players over the course of a season conducted by Bolonchuk and Lukaski[14] arrived at dissimilar results. There was a decrease in endomorphy, an increase in mesomorphy, and no change in ectomorphy. Similar results were also found in an evolutionary study on rugby players by Olds.[53] There was an increase in mesomorphy and decreases in endomorphy and ectomorphy.

BODY SIZE AND BODY PROPORTIONS

Although body type and somatotype rating systems were essential to the study of human morphological measurement, they were nevertheless criticized by researchers in the field, both in theory and practice. In theory, researchers were critical of the preconceived dichotomous types selected to determine physique; in practice, criticism was directed at the deductive subjectivity of the designated methods and processes utilized.[62] In order to objectively study the body size and body proportions inherent in physique variations, inductive anthropometric ratios and indices were used as methods of assessment (Table 2.4).[41,43,71–73]

FACTOR TYPES

The study of factor types through the use of factor analysis was first investigated by Spearman,[68] and later by Rees and Eysenck[61] and Thurstone.[75] Rees and Eysenck[61] and Rees,[59,60] in studies of 200 men and 200 women, intercorrelated and factor-analyzed 18 anthropometric measurements obtained from the subjects. The predominant factors found were those of height and chest breadth for men, and height, symphysis height, and hip and chest circumferences for women. The male measures were determined through a ratio formulation, whereas the female measures were calculated through the use of a regression equation. Results from both systems were plotted on normal curves relative to mean scores and standard deviation units. From these figures, body types were formed to reflect two-dimensional rectangular classifications. Euromorphy was exemplified by large breadth and circumference measures relative to length, mesomorphy by the intermediate relationship between laterality and linearity, and leptomorphy by small breadth and circumference ratings relative to length.

Thurstone,[75] in his study of factory types, intercorrelated 12 anthropometric measures taken from his sample subjects and found four primary factor loadings. They were head, trunk, girth, and extremity sizes. In their study of psychotic patients, Moore and Hsu[50] factor-analyzed 31 measures of the head and body. Four factors were found: (1) general body size, (2) length, (3) lateral, and (4) circumference measures. Similarly Burt,[15,16] in his investigation of the body builds of British children and adults, found general body size, length, breadth, girth, and weight to be the prominent factors. Howells[41] also reported high-factor loadings on size, length, breadth, girth, and weight.

Factor analytical methods of study enabled investigators in the field to develop statistical body-build indices that were objectively determined. These indices represented factor types that described the morphological makeup (size and shape) of the body in qualitative anthropological relationships.[19]

TABLE 2.4
Factor Analysis Summary

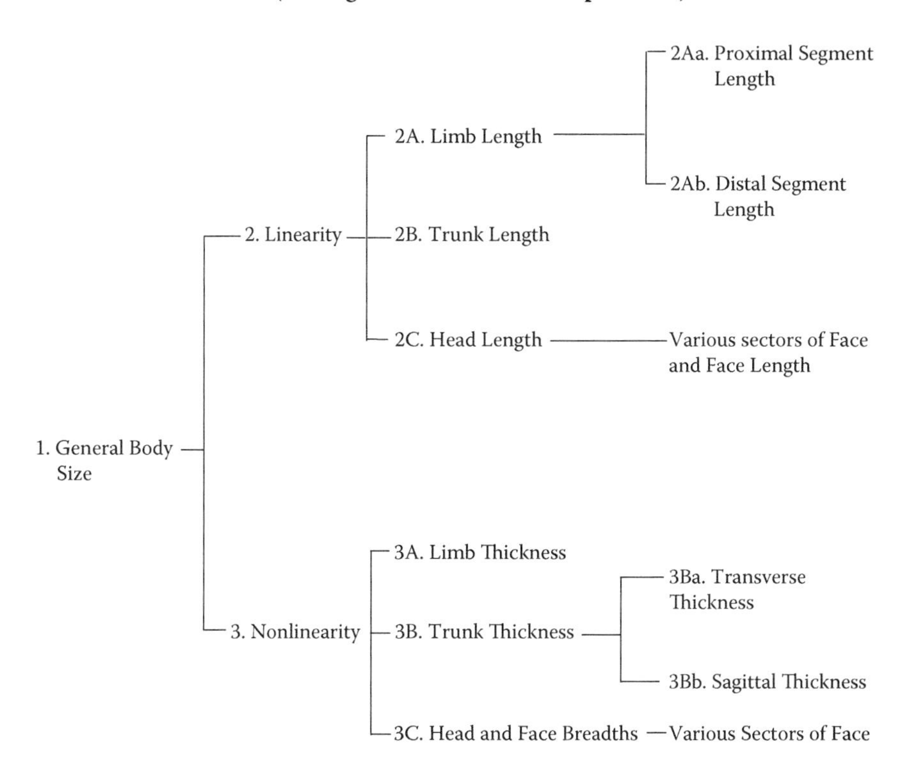

Source: Adapted from Tanner, J.M., in *Anthropology Today: An Encyclopedic Inventory,* Kroeber, A.L., Ed., The University of Chicago Press, Chicago, p.762, 1953. With permission of the publisher.

DYSPLASIA TYPE INDICES

Dysplasia type indices have also been useful in study of bodily disharmony or dysplasia relative to structural deviation from established norms of physique assessment. Kretschmer,[44] Viola,[77] and Sheldon et al.[63] developed classification systems for such study. Kretschmer[44] believed dysplasia or structural disharmony to be reflective of body type extremes. His assessment for such study was anthroposcopic in method and was determined through the study of bodily features relative to high-profile angularity, athletic sturdiness, or asthenic emaciation in the pyknic, athletic, and asthenic body types, respectively. Viola[77] defined dysplasia as the structural disharmony of body parts. Based on index measurements of trunk volume and extremity length, Viola designated disharmonic types through the assessment of the sum of the particular deviations in terms of percentages taken from the total average of the measurements obtained. Sheldon et al.[63] defined dysplasia as the inconsistent or disproportionate mixtures of endomorphy, mesomorphy, and ectomorphy in designated regions of the body. Each of these regions was separately somatotyped. Dysplasia was calculated through the assessment of the sums of the differences between each of the regional components, which were then totaled to form the final dysplasia figure. This figure was then compared to developed population norms.

Although the study of factor types and dysplasia types advanced the theoretical and practical knowledge and application parameters of body-build research, criticisms were nevertheless directed at such study. Sills,[64] in this regard, reported that the utilization of a few body measures did not satisfactorily provide pertinent and essential anthropometric data. Domey et al.,[25] in their overview of body-build rating systems, designated that such morphological indices provided only basic data results, which limited the effectiveness of such systems for the adequate assessment of body build.

BODY-BUILD INDICES

Recent typological systems of dysplasia can be described as index oriented, utilizing anthropometric measures of selective representative landmarks (height, weight, and body lengths, breadths, and circumferences) in the determination of body size and body proportionality.[47] Hirata[36,37] developed a stout–lean F-index rating system based on height and weight ratios, typing athletes along vertically and horizontally plotted axes and demonstrating their tallness, shortness, stoutness, and leanness in comparison to average body-build measures. Behnke[8,9] classified the structural bodily deviations of athletes from designated norm girth landmark measures through somatogram line representations of body size and shape.[42] Dupertuis[26] formulated a structural profile based on representative length and breadth skeletal measures of body landmarks through the use of percentage breadth/height ratio deviations from calculated group norm values plotted on graph evaluation forms. Battinelli[6,7] categorized structural variational differences through the formulation of breadth–length–upper–lower body classifications of morphological disharmonies relative to types (direction) and subtypes (extent) (Figure 2.4 and Appendix 2).[4,7] Katch[42,49] formulated a body profile in which muscular and nonmuscular proportionality deviations from given reference constants were measured to form a ponderal somatogram (Figure 2.5). The muscular variables included the shoulders, chest, biceps, forearm, thigh, and calf circumferences, while the nonmuscular girth measures were taken from the abdomen, hips, knee, wrist, and ankle. The body profile was based on Behnke's original somatogram and extended to form a ponderal somatogram which differentiates muscular body areas from nonmuscular segments and then compares them as body mass equivalents.[42,48,49]

BODY-BUILD INDICES AND BIOMECHANICS

The physique components of body size and body proportions can, in essence, enhance or limit physical performance.[1,9,11,12,30–32,36,37,39,69,72,73,79,83] Large and heavy-

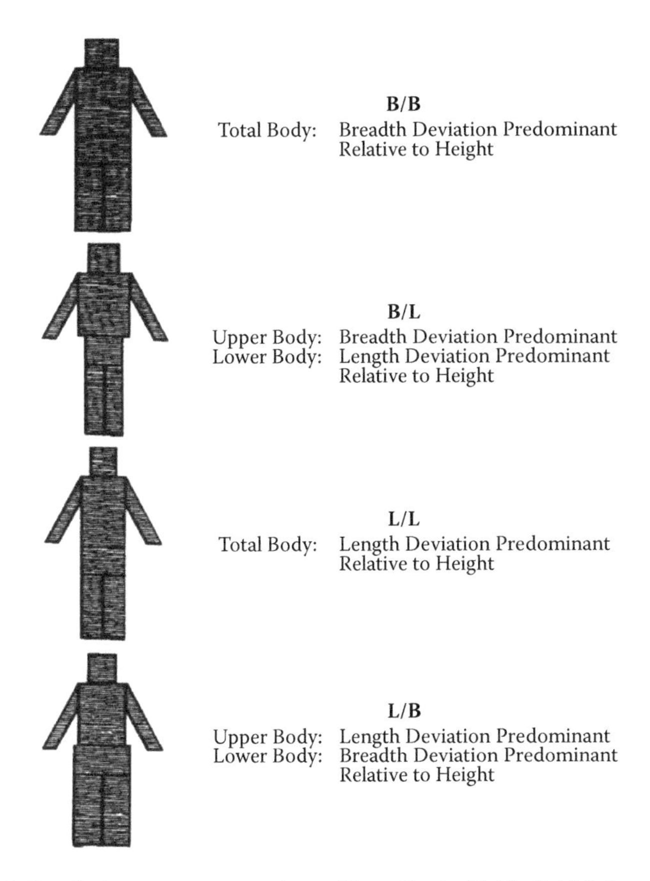

FIGURE 2.4 Dysplasia type representations. (From Battinelli, T., *British Journal of Sports Medicine*, 18, 22–25, 1984. With permission from the BMJ Publishing Group.)

bodied athletes may have a significant advantage over their smaller and lighter-weighted counterparts in reference to sports activities where the magnitude of force is used to overcome the resistive stability of another. Similarly, weight may play a role in propulsive activities against the reactive resistance of the environment. Smaller and lighter athletes may be better predisposed to activities demanding quick movement acceleration and continued motion over periods of time. Smaller athletes would also possess higher strength-to-mass ratios than do larger athletes.

In reference to body proportions, taller athletes with longer limbs may have a biomechanical advantage over shorter participants with shorter limbs relative to activities that are power oriented. The shorter athletes with shorter limbs would have the advantage in activities where speed generation and rotational abilities are mandated. The higher center of gravity in taller athletes would also be advantageous in activities that involve the vertical and horizontal explosive power exhibited in jumping. Shorter individuals with a lower center of gravity would possess a greater amount of stability. Shorter athletes may also have an advantage over their taller counterparts

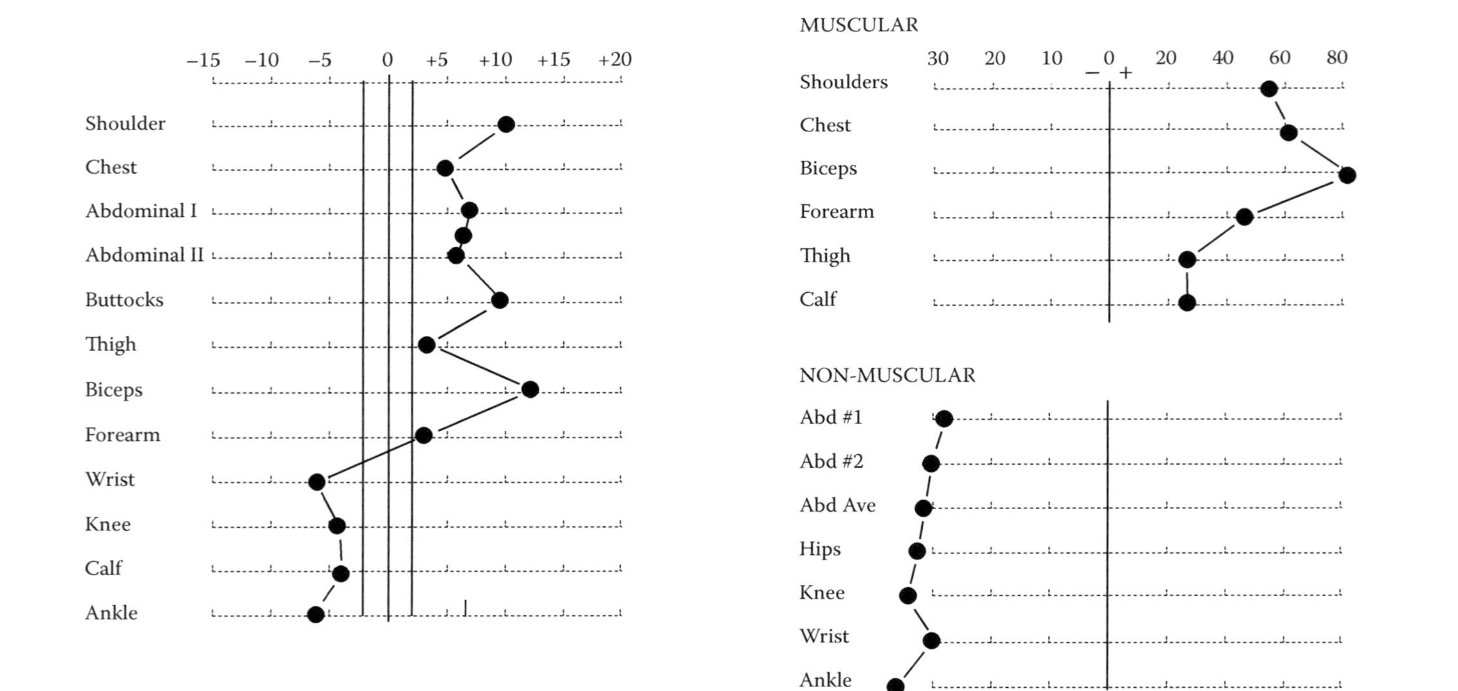

FIGURE 2.5 Original and ponderal somatograms; deviations from given norm values. (Reprinted with permission from Katch, F.I., in *Body Composition and Physical Performance*, Marriott, B.M. and J. Grumstrup-Scott, Eds., National Academy Press, Washington, DC, 1992. Copyright 1992 by the National Academy of Sciences. Courtesy of the National Academy Press, Washington, DC.)

in the execution of weight training patterns of motion. The weight resistance would be lifted through a shorter distance, thereby exerting force over a shorter distance.

BODY-BUILD INDICES AND PHYSICAL PERFORMANCE

Unlike somatotype-oriented systems of classification, body-build indices are generally computed from ratios of two or more body measures that demonstrate the size and proportional differences of body parts from one another relative to representative average norms. The body measures usually include height, weight, lengths, breadths, and circumferences.[12,46]

Body size and body proportionality studies of Olympic, champion athletes, and athletes have been demonstrative of the physique similarities and dissimilarities, individually and collectively, for both men and women, associated with given athletic activities.[1,8,9,17,23,25,31,36,37,39,40,48,49,51,53,59,64,69,72,73]

1. Sprinters were short and muscular.
2. Distance runners were small and lean.
3. Throwers were tall and heavy bodied.
4. Basketball and volleyball players were tall and lean.
5. Cyclists and soccer participants were small and stout.
6. Hurdlers, swimmers, and high jumpers were large and lean.
7. Rowers were heavy in weight and tall in height.
8. Gymnasts were light in weight and short in height with short arms and legs.
9. Weight lifters were excessively muscular.
10. Football players were large and muscular.
11. Defensive hockey players were taller and heavier than their offensive forward counterparts.
12. Figure skaters were small, lean, and somewhat muscular.
13. Speed skaters were similar in height to soccer players, skiers, distance runners, and weight lifters, but shorter than basketball players, football players, track and field athletes, and swimmers.
14. Rugby players were tall and heavy.

SUMMARY

In summary, the conclusions that can be drawn from these studies indicated that:

1. Physique classification systems generally measure size, shape, and form through anthroposcopic and anthropometric methods of evaluation.
2. The somatotypes of athletes within given sports activities, although similar to some extent, were dissimilar relative to size and proportions within given events and positional play.
3. The somatotypes of champion athletes were progressively more similar, relative to size and proportions, as competitive levels increased in regard to given sports activities and to given events and positional play.

4. Mesomorphs were found to be superior to their endomorphic and ectomorphic counterparts in terms of strength, speed, agility, and endurance.
5. Middle and distance runners were found to be classified within moderate ranges of mesomorphy and ectomorphy, while strength- and speed-dependent athletes tended to be ranked high in mesomorphy and low in ectomorphy.
6. Changes in somatotype due to training and competitive sport participation over a period of time may or may not occur.
7. Male athletes were more mesomorphic, but less endomorphic and ectomorphic, than their female counterparts.
8. In reference to the male athletes, weight lifters were more endomorphic and mesomorphic, but less ectomorphic, than were the boxers and judo competitors. Gymnasts and canoeists were more mesomorphic and less endomorphic than were the fencers, field hockey players, cyclists, and rowers.
9. In reference to the somatotypes of female athletes, gymnasts and track and field athletes were less endomorphic than were the canoeists, rowers, and swimmers.
10. Factor types and dysplasia types have been used to study physique variations through analytical and statistical methods of assessment.
11. Body size and body proportions can influence (enhance/limit) physical performance capabilities.
12. Structural deviations from designated norm values relative to body build may differ among athletes of selective sports activities.
13. Large and heavy-bodied athletes may have a significant advantage over smaller and lighter-weighted counterparts in reference to physical activities where the magnitude of force is used to overcome the resistive stability of another.
14. Smaller and lighter athletes may be better predisposed to activities demanding quick movement acceleration and continued motion over periods of time.
15. Taller athletes with longer limbs and a higher center of gravity may have a biomechanical advantage over shorter participants with shorter limbs relative to activities that are power oriented.
16. Shorter athletes with shorter limbs and a lower center of gravity would have greater stability and a greater advantage in activities where speed generation and rotational abilities are mandated.
17. Body size and body proportionality studies of Olympic, champion athletes, and athletes have been demonstrative of the physique similarities and dissimilarities, individually and collectively, for both men and women indigenous to given athletic activities.

GLOSSARY

Anthropometric somatotype Physique rating component system of live body measurement classification
Anthropometry Quantitative measures of selected human landmarks
Anthroposcopy Visual study of bodily features and form
Apoplectic habitus Heavy and solid physique
Asthenic Physique predominance of body length relative to breadth and circumference
Athletic Physique predominance of muscularity
Body build Physique
Body-build indices Ratios of two or more body measures that demonstrate the size and proportional differences of body parts from one another relative to representative average norms
Body size The physical height and mass or weight of the body
Body type Physique rating type system of classification
Dysplasia/disproportions Variational body regional differences in physique rating relative to given norm ranges
Ectodermal layer Embryonic germ layer of skin- and nervous-system-related areas of the body
Ectomorphy Somatotype predominance of linearity and fragility
Endodermal layer Embryonic germ layer source of visceral and fat related areas of the body
Endomorphy Somatotype predominance of roundness and softness
Euromorphy Body-build predominance of breadth relative to height
Factor types The body-build variables or types that have been identified and quantified
Leptomorphy Body-build predominance of height relative to breadth
Macrosplanchnic Large heavy trunk and short-limbed body build
Mesodermal layer Embryonic germ layer source of muscle, connective tissue, and bone-related areas of the body
Mesomorphy Somatotype predominance of squareness and hardness or intermediate height and breadth
Microsplanchnic Small trunk and long-limbed body build
Morphology The study of human form and structure
Normosplanchnic Medium trunk and medium-limbed body build
Pyknic Corpulent body build
Somatogram/structural profile Representative depictions of body regional deviations from given norm ranges
Somatotype Physique rating component system of classification
Type cerebral Vertical-related physique
Type digestif Visceral-related physique
Type musculaire Muscular-related physique

REFERENCES

1. Abernathy, B. et al., *The Biophysical Foundations of Human Movement,* 2nd ed., Human Kinetics Publishers, Champaign, IL, 2005.
2. Adams, W.C., *Foundations of Physical Education, Exercise, and Sport Sciences,* Lea and Febiger, Philadelphia, 1991.
3. Astrand, P. et al., *Textbook of Work Physiology: Physiological Basis of Exercise,* 4th ed., Human Kinetics Publishers, Champaign, IL, 2003.
4. Bale, P., *The Somatotypes of Sportsmen and Sportswomen,* Brighton Polytechnic, Chelsea School of Human Movement, 1984.
5. Barrow, H.M. and J.P. Brown, *Man and Movement: Principles of Physical Education,* 4th ed., Lea and Febiger, Philadelphia, 1988.
6. Battinelli, T., A simplistic approach to structural dysplasia assessment: description and validation, *British Journal of Sports Medicine*, 18, 22–25, 1984.
7. Battinelli, T., Constitutional disharmony and selected components of motor ability, *Human Biology*, 48, 465–474, 1976.
8. Behnke, A.R., Physique and exercise, in *Exercise Physiology,* Behnke, A.R., Ed., Academic Press, New York, pp. 359–385, 1968.
9. Behnke, A.R. and J. Royce, Body size, shape, and composition of several types of athletes, *Journal of Sports Medicine and Physical Fitness*, 6, 75–88, 1966.
10. Beunen, G. and J. Borms, Kinanthropometry: roots, developments and future, *Journal of Sports Sciences*, 8, 1–15, 1990.
11. Bloomfield, J., T.R. Ackland, and B.C. Elliott, *Applied Anatomy and Biomechanics in Sport,* Blackwell Scientific Publications, Boston, 1994.
12. Boileau, R.A. and C.A. Horswill, Body composition in sports: measurement and applications for weight loss and gain, in *Exercise and Sport Science,* Garrett, W.E., Jr. and D.T. Kirkendall, Eds., Lippincott Williams, and Wilkins, Philadelphia, 2000.
13. Boileau, R.A., and T.G. Lohman, The measurement of human physique and its effect on physical performance, *Orthopedic Clinics of North America*, 7, 563–581, 1977.
14. Bolonchuk, W.W., and H.C. Lukaski, Changes in somatotype and body composition of college football players over a season, *Journal of Sports Medicine*, 27, 247–251, 1987.
15. Burt, C., A comparison of factor analysis and analysis of variance, *British Journal of Psychology*, 1, 3–26, 1947.
16. Burt, C., The factorial study of physical types, *Man*, 82–86, 1944.
17. Carter, J.E.L., Somatotypes of athletes, *Human Biology*, 42, 535–569, 1970.
18. Carter, J.E.L., *The Heath–Carter Somatotype Method,* 3rd ed., San Diego State University, San Diego, CA, 1980.
19. Carter, J.E.L., and B.H. Heath, *Somatotyping-Development Applications,* Cambridge University Press, Cambridge, 1990.
20. Carter, J.E.L. and R.H. Rahe, Effects of stressful underwater demolition training on body structure, *Medicine and Science in Sports*, 7, 304–308, 1975.
21. Carter, J.E.L. and W.H. Phillips, Structural changes in exercising middle-aged males during a two year period, *Journal of Applied Physiology*, 27, 787–794, 1969.
22. Carter, J.E.L., S.P. Rubrey, and D.R. Sleet, Somatotypes of Montreal Olympic Athletes, *Medicine and Science in Sports*, 16, 53–88, 1982.
23. Cureton, T.K., *Physical Fitness of Champion Athletes,* The University of Illinois Press, Urbana, 1951.
24. de Garay, A., L. Levine, and J.E.L. Carter, *Genetic and Anthropological Studies of Olympic Athletes,* Academic Press, New York, 1974.

25. Domey, R.G., J.E. Duckworth, and A.J. Morandi, Taxonomies and correlates of physique, *Psychological Bulletin*, 62, 411–436, 1964.
26. Dupertuis, C.W. The structural profile, *American Journal of Physical Anthropology*, 41, 476, 1974.
27. Foley, J.P., S.R. Bird, and J.A. White, Anthropometric comparison of cyclists from different events, *British Journal of Sports Medicine*, 23, 30–33, 1989.
28. Fox, E.I., R.W. Bowers, and M.L. Foss, *The Physiological Basis for Exercise and Sport,* 5th ed., Brown and Benchmark, Madison, WI, 1993.
29. Gay, L.R. *Educational Research: Competencies for Analysis and Application,* 5th ed., Prentice Hall, Englewood Cliffs, NJ, 1996.
30. Gualdi-Russo, E. and L. Zaccagni, Somaotype, role and performance in elite volleyball players, *Journal of Sports Medicine and Physical Fitness,* 41, 256–262, 2001.
31. Harman, E.A. and P.N. Frykman, The relationship of body size and composition to the performance of physically demanding tasks, in *Body Composition and Physical Performance,* Marriott, B.M. and J. Grumstrup-Scott, Eds., National Academy Press, Washington, DC, 1992.
32. Harman, E.A., The biomechanics of resistance exercise, in *Essentials of Strength Training and Conditioning,* 2nd ed., Baechle, T.R. and R.W. Earle, Eds., Human Kinetics Publishers, Champaign, IL, 2000.
33. Heath, B.H. and J.E.L. Carter, A comparison of somatotype methods, *American Journal of Physical Anthropology*, 27, 87–99, 1966.
34. Heath, B.H. and J.E.L. Carter, A modified somatotype method, *American Journal of Physical Anthropology*, 27, 57–74, 1967.
35. Hebbelink, M. et al., Anthropometric of characteristics of female Olympic rowers, *Canadian Journal of Applied Sport Servies,* 5, 255–262, 1980.
36. Hirata, K., Physique and age of Tokyo Olympic champions, *Journal of Sports Medicine and Physical Fitness*, 6, 107–222, 1966.
37. Hirata, K., *The Evaluating Method of Physique and Physical Fitness and Its Practical Application*, Hirata Institute, Gifu Prefecture, Japan, 1964.
38. Hollings, S.C. and G.J. Robson, A profile of New Zealand elite rowers, *New Zealand Journal of Sports Medicine*, 20, 2–5, Summer, 1992.
39. Holloway, J.B., Individual differences and their implications for resistance training, in *Essentials of Strength Training and Conditioning*, 2nd ed., Baechle, T.R. and R.W. Earle, Eds., Human Kinetics Publishers, Champaign, IL, 2000.
40. Houston, M.E. and H.J. Green, Physiological and anthropometric characteristics of elite Canadian ice hockey players, *American Journal of Sports Medicine*, 16, 123–128, 1976.
41. Howells, W.W., Factors of human physique, *American Journal of Physical Anthropology*, 9, 159–191, 1951.
42. Katch, F.I., New approaches to body composition evaluation and some relationships to dynamic muscular strength, in *Body Composition and Physical Performance,* Marriott, B.M. and J. Grumstrup-Scott, Eds., National Academy Press, Washington, DC, 1992.
43. Kerr, D. and T. Ackland, Kinantropometry: physique assessment of the athlete, in *Clinical Sports Nutrition,* 2nd ed., Burke, L. and V. Deakin, Eds., McGraw-Hill Companies, Australia, 2000.
44. Kretschmer, E., *Physique and Character* (Sprott, W.J.H., trans), Harcourt, Brace and Company, New York, 1925.
45. Leake, C.N. and J.E.L. Carter, Comparison of body composition and somatotype of trained female triathletes, *Journal of Sports Sciences*, 9, 125–135, 1991.

46. LeVeau, B., T. Ward, and R.C. Nelson, Body dimensions of Japanese and American gymnasts, *Medicine and Science in Sports*, 6, 146–150, 1974.
47. Malina, R.M., Anthropometry, in *Physiological Assessment of Human Fitness*, Maud, P.J. and C. Foster, Eds., Human Kinetics Publishers, Champaign, IL, 1995.
48. McArdle, W.D., F.I. Katch, and V.L. Katch, *Sports and Exercise Nutrition,* 2nd ed., Lippincott, Williams, and Wilkins, Philadelphia, 2004.
49. McArdle, W.D., F.I. Katch, and V.L. Katch, *Exercise Physiology: Energy, Nutrition, and Human Performance,* 5th ed., Lippincott, Williams and Wilkins, Baltimore, MD, 2001.
50. Moore, T.V. and E.H. Hsu, Factorial analysis of anthropological measurements in psychotic patients, *Human Biology*, 18, 133–157, 1946.
51. Morehouse, L.E. and P.J. Rasch, *Sports Medicine for Trainers,* W.B. Saunders, Philadelphia, 1964.
52. Norgan, N.G., Anthropometry and physical performance, in *Anthropometry: The Individual and the Population,* Ulijaszek, S.J. and C.G.N. Mascie-Taylor, Eds., Cambridge University Press, London, 1994.
53. Olds, T., The evolution of physique in male rugby players in the twentieth century, *Journal of Sport Sciences,* 19, 253–262, 2001.
54. Orvanova, E., Somatotypes of weight lifters, *Journal of Sports Sciences*, 8, 119–137, 1990.
55. Parnell, R.W., *Behavior and Physique,* Edward Arnold Publisher, London, 1958.
56. Pollock, M.L., C. Foster, J. Anholm, J. Hare, P. Farrell, M. Maksud, and A.S. Jackson, Body composition of Olympic speed skating candidates, *Research Quarterly for Exercise and Sport*, 53, 150–155, 1982.
57. Powers, S.K. and E.T. Howley, *Exercise Physiology: Theory and Application to Fitness and Performance,* Brown and Benchmark, Dubuque, IA, 1990.
58. Powers, S.K. and E.T. Howley, *Exercise Physiology: Theory and Application to Fitness and Performance,* 2nd ed., Brown and Benchmark, Dubuque, IA, 1994.
59. Rees, L., A factorial study of physical constitution in women, *Journal of Mental Science*, 96, 620–632, 1950.
60. Rees, L., Constitutional factors and abnormal behavior, in *Handbook of Abnormal Psychology,* Eysenck, H., Ed., Basic Books, New York, 1960.
61. Rees, L. and H.J. Eysenck, A factorial study of some morphological and psychological aspects of human constitution, *Journal of Mental Science*, 91, 8, 1945.
62. Ross, W.D. et al., Somatotypes of Canadian figure skaters, *American Journal of Sports Medicine*, 17, 195–205, 1977.
63. Sheldon, W.H., S.S. Stevens, and W.B. Tucker, *The Varieties of Human Physique,* Harper and Brothers, New York, 1940.
64. Sills, F.D., Anthropometry in relation to physical education, in *Science and Medicine of Exercise and Sport,* 2nd ed., Johnson, W.R. and E.R. Buskirk, Eds., Harper & Row, New York, pp. 24–33, 1974.
65. Sills, F.D. and J. Mitchem, Prediction of performance on performance on physical fitness tests by means of somatotype rating, *Research Quarterly*, 24, 64–71, 1957.
66. Sills, F.D. and P.W. Everett, The relationship of extreme somatotypes to performance in motor and strength tests, *Research Quarterly*, 24, 223–228, 1953.
67. Simon, E., Morphological development and functional efficiency, in *International Research in Sport and Physical Education,* Jokl, E. and E. Simon, Eds., Charles C. Thomas, Springfield, IL, 1964.
68. Spearman, C., *Abilities of Man,* Macmillan, Condon, 1927.

69. Spence, D.E. et al., Description profiles of highly skilled women volleyball players, *Medicine and Science in Sports*, 20, 299–302, 1980.
70. Stepnicka, J., *Typological and Motor Characteristics of Athletes and University Students,* Prague, Charles University, 1972.
71. Swain, D.P., The influence of body mass in endurance bicycling, *Medicine and Science in Sport and Exercise*, 26, 58–63, 1994.
72. Tanner, J.M., Growth and constitution, *Anthropology Today,* Kroeber, A.L., Ed., University of Chicago Press, Chicago, 1951.
73. Tanner, J.M., *The Physique of the Olympic Athlete*, Allen and Unwin, London, 1964.
74. Tucker, W.B. and W.A. Lessa, Man: a constitutional investigation, *The Quarterly Review of Biology*, 15, 411–456, 1940.
75. Thurstone, L.L. Factor analysis and body types, *Psychometrika*, 1, 15–22, 1946.
76. Van Huss, et al., *Physical Activity in Modern Living,* 2nd ed., Prentice-Hall, Englewood Cliffs, NJ, 1969.
77. Viola, G., Il Mio Metodo Di Valutazione Della Constituzione Individuale, *Endocrinologia e Patologia Costituzionale*, 12, 387–480, 1937.
78. Willgoose, E.E., *Evaluation in Health Education and Physical Education*, McGraw-Hill, New York, 1961.
79. Wilmore, J.H., Sports medicine, in *Anthropometric Standardization Reference Manual*, Lohman, T.G., A.E. Roche, and R. Martorell, Eds., Human Kinetics Publishers, Champaign, IL, 1988.
80. Wilmore, J.H., and D.L. Costell, *Physiology of Sport and Exercise*, Human Kinetics Publishers, Champaign, IL, 1994.
81. Wilmore, J.H., C.H. Brown, and J.A. Davis, Body physique and composition of the female distance runner, *Annals of the New York Academy of Science*, 301, 764–776, 1977.
82. Wilmore, J.H. et al., Athletic profile of professional football players, *Physician and Sports Medicine*, 4, 54–54, 1976.
83. Withers, R., N.P. Craig, and K.I. Norton, Somatotypes of South Australian male athletes, *Human Biology*, 58, 337–356, 1986.
84. Withers, R. et al., Somatotypes of South Australian female games players, *Human Biology*, 59, 575–589, 1987.

3 Body Fat and Fat-Free Composition

INTRODUCTION

While body-build indices enabled investigators to basically study the general body size and body mass of athletes and nonathletes, the information derived from such studies was limited relative to tissue composition. Cureton[16] indicated that, although individuals of a given height could have similar weights, they could still differ in proportions of bone, muscle, and fat. Limitations of this nature relative to height–weight measures were demonstrated by Behnke et al.[6,85] They reported that excessive weight for height and age could be regarded erroneously as obesity. By determining the specific gravity of football players who ranged in weight from 170 to 260 pounds, they found that 11 of 17 overweight players were classified within low-fat categories. Keys and Brozek[42] corroborated these results; they found subjects to be misclassified by insurance scales when measured through body composition methods of evaluation.

DIRECT AND INDIRECT METHODS OF MEASURE

Body composition analysis of the fat and lean components of the body can be determined through direct and indirect methods of measure (Table 3.1 and Table 3.2) Direct methods of measure have been based on the study of the chemical and physical analysis of cadavers relative to the body constituents of fat, water, protein, and minerals.[9,19,50,52,57,83] These analytic systems of measure have set the norm standards within which live-body measurements determined through indirect assessment can be made. Indirect methods include: densitometric, dilutional, nitrogen, potassium, x-ray, ultrasound, and anthropometric measures of the body as well as some of the newer techniques in use today, such as computed tomography, magnetic resonance, electrical conductivity, infrared interactance, photon absorptiometry, and air displacement pletysmography. These methods provide a noninvasive assessment of fat and fat-free tissue. Densitometry or underwater weighing has become the indirect norm standard for purposes of significant comparison. However, while these systems can accurately and reliably measure body composition, some drawbacks remain relative to cost, administrative feasibility, time, possible radiation exposure, and general population applicability.[36,57,81]

TABLE 3.1
Body Composition Measurement

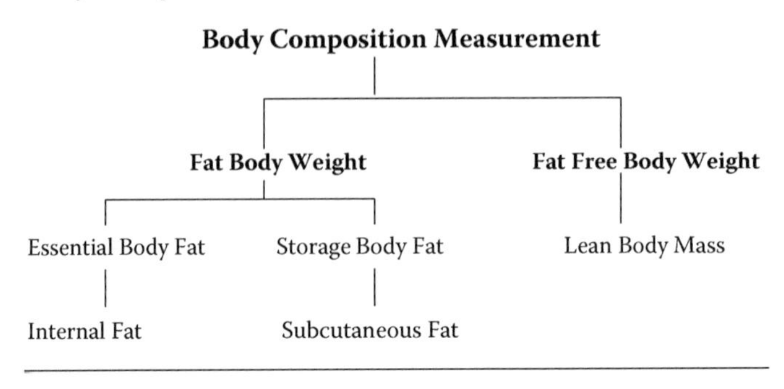

TABLE 3.2

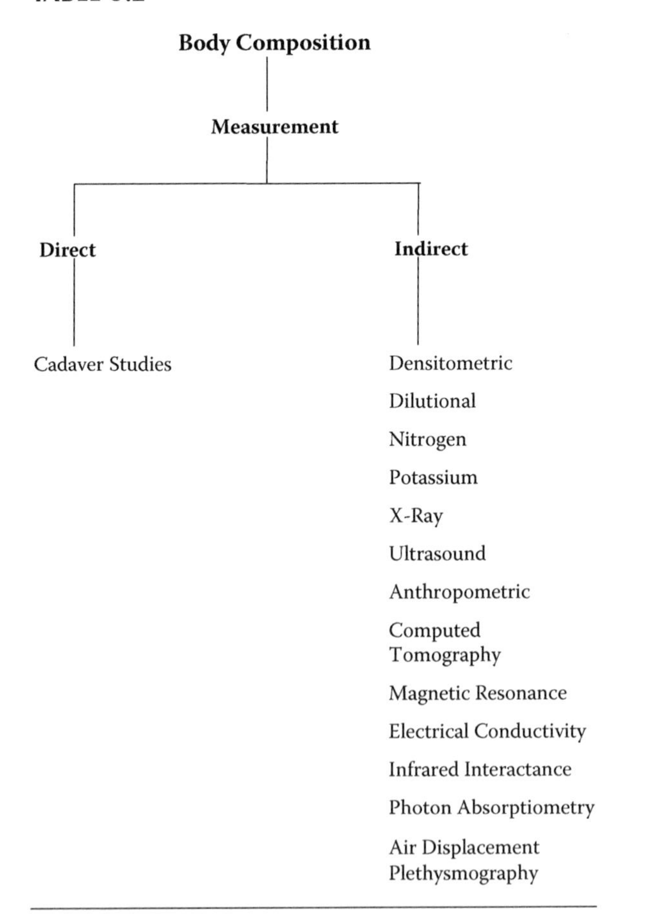

DENSITOMETRY AND HYDROMETRY

The densitometric measurement of the body utilizing the underwater weighing procedures originally developed by Archimedes can generally be described as the determination of specific gravity and body density through water volume displacement of weight in air and weight in water.[14,25,30,81,88] Body density values can then be converted to fat and fat-free tissue formulations. Hydrometric methods of measure incorporate the use of isotopic deuterium and tritium oxide dilutions for the estimation of total body water. Infrared spectrographic procedures and scintillation counters are utilized for assessment purposes through the measurement of total body water so that lean body mass can be estimated.[73]

TOTAL NITROGEN AND TOTAL BODY POTASSIUM

Total body nitrogen can be measured through neutron activation analysis of bodily emitted gamma rays. Nitrogen levels can be quantified by such analysis, enabling researchers to determine the amount of protein in muscle and nonmuscle tissue body compartments through equation calculations. Similarly, total body potassium is also measured through gamma ray bodily emissions for the chemical determination of body cell mass relative to fat and fat-free tissue.[10,14,16,38,39,43,46,47,52,70] High potassium contents are indicative of little fat tissue in the body.

COMPUTED TOMOGRAPHY AND MAGNETIC RESONANCE

Bone, muscle, and fat can be measured through x-ray methods. While the conversion of x-ray-measured skinfold thickness to estimations of body fat has been a problem, recent advances in radiographic techniques have provided the quantitative information needed.[4] Two new scanning methods of fat measurement currently in use are those of computed tomography and magnetic resonance. Through the use of x-ray beam and magnetic scanning procedures, radiographic cross images of essential and storage fat are produced, enabling investigators to measure body tissue composition.[10,32,52,58] Both methodologies assess fat and fat-free tissue differences through formula estimations of the volume and density of the generated body images.

ELECTRICAL CONDUCTIVITY AND ULTRASOUND

Body electrical conductivity and bioelectrical impedance are based on the principle that lean tissue has a higher electrolyte content than does fat tissue and is, therefore, more conductive electrically in this regard.[10,31,48,52,53,67,68,88] In electrical conductivity analysis, an overall body covering instrument constructed around a solenoidal coil is used, through which electromagnetic radiation can measure the coil impedance changes (full to empty) that take place (Figure 3.1). The reactive/resistance tissue differences in electrical flow can be quantified through calculative formulas, making it possible for fat and fat-free tissue levels to be determined.[45] Bioelectric impedance

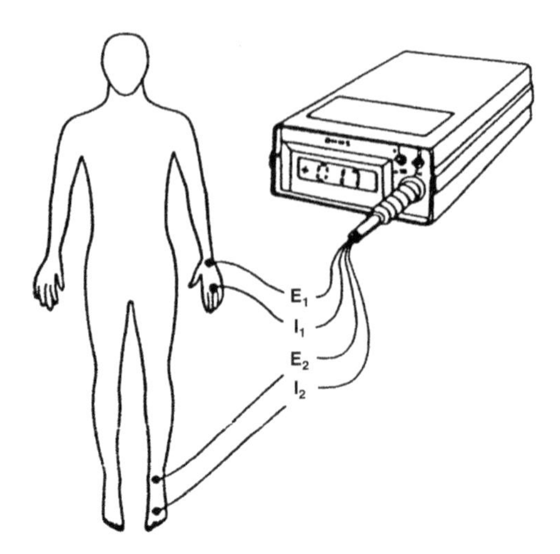

FIGURE 3.1 Representative diagram of bioelectric impedance measurement. (From Lucaski, H. C. et al. Assessment of fat free mass using bioelectric impedance measurements of the human body. *American Journal of Clinical Nutrition*, 41: 810–817, 1985. Reproduced with permission from The American Journal of Clinical Nutrition.)

measurement is also based on the electrical flow resistance through lean and fat tissue. Electrodes placed on the hands and feet are used to measure the flow impedance.[52,72] The flow impedance values are then translated into body density formularization from which fat and fat-free tissue ratios can be determined. Both of these methods can be affected by total body water levels; therefore, water balance should be maintained in order to validly assess fat content.[39,88] Low body water levels may be indicative of lower fat percentage estimates.

Both methodologies assess fat and fat-free tissue differences through formula estimations of the volume and density of the generated body images. Similarly, ultrasound methods of measurement have also been used in the assessment of body composition components. Since bone, muscle, and fat have different density levels, high frequency sound waves can be used to identify and quantify different tissue types.[4,10,14,23] Sound waves produced by transducers pass through body tissue and are reflected by different density levels of electrical amplification impulses. Tissue thickness can be calculated with the use of electronic calipers.

INFRARED INTERACTANCE AND PHOTON ABSORPTIOMETRY

Probably two of the newer methods of measuring body composition are those of infrared interactance and dual body photon absorptiometry. Infrared interactance employs the use of an electromagnetic radiation body probe to measure the absorptive and reflective spectrographic chemical properties of fat, water, and protein.[32,52,81,88] Since the absorptive and reflective properties of these tissues differ, the fat and fat-free ratios can be quantified and determined. In reference to photon absorptiometry, two-energy-level photon scans are made of the body. The energy level absorptive ratio differences that are observed are used to determine the bone mineral mass and the fat and fat-free soft tissue compositional amounts.[10,14,36,57]

AIR DISPLACEMENT PLETHYSMOGRAPHY: BODY POD

Body Pod methodology is based on the volume measure of the bodily displacement of air relative to pressure gradient differences.[15,52,81,83] The Bod Pod consists of one chamber partitioned into two sections. The subject would sit in the pod for a brief period of time while the air volume displacement is assessed by diaphragmatic gauged movement pressure changes. Formulas are then utilized to calculate the body composition measures of fat and fat-free ratios. As a recent entry into the field of body composition, air displacement plethysmography has become a significant method of assessment.[52]

ANTHROPOMETRIC METHODS OF MEASURE

Although different and newer methods have made inroads in the analysis of body composition, anthropometry has remained the most prevalent and practical indirect measure. In general, anthropometric assessments of fat and fat-free tissue have been determined through the use of skeletal diameters, skinfolds, and circumferences as methods of measure relative to established body-density norms (Table 3.3).[57,59]

In reference to skeletal diameter studies, Van Dobeln[80] developed fat-free weight formulations through the measurement of height, wrist breadth, and knee breadth. Behnke[3,28] utilized 12 bone-breadth measures in relation to height and weight in his development of quantitative formulas for the assessment of lean body weight and percentage of body fat. Wilmore and Behnke[87] simplified this method of measure in a subsequent study. Four bone diameters were measured instead of 12, and the

TABLE 3.3

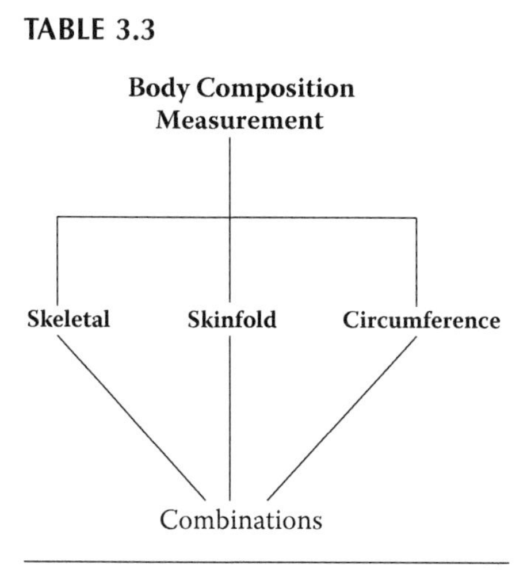

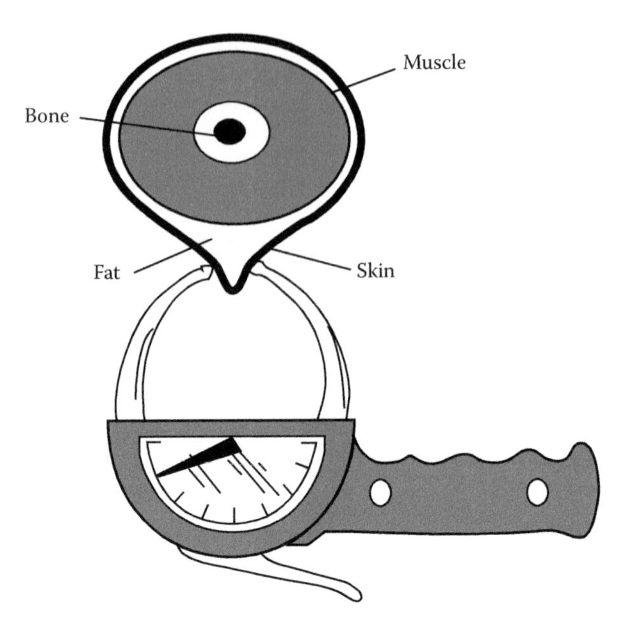

FIGURE 3.2 Fat skinfold drawing. (From Williams, M., *Nutrition for Fitness and Sport*, 4th ed., McGraw-Hill, New York, 1995. Reproduced with the permission of the McGraw-Hill Companies.)

calculative results were significantly related to Behnke's earlier and more comprehensive method of measure.

Lean body weight and percentage of body fat have also been measured through the use of skinfold measurements in relation to established body density norms (Figure 3.2).[83] Matiegka[51] was probably the first to develop an equation for the calculation of body fat using surface area and skinfold measurements. Edwards,[20] in his study of body composition, evaluated repeated skinfold measures taken from approximately 50 landmark sites and demonstrated a variational relationship of body weight to skinfold thickness. Brozek[11] and Brozek and Keys[12] were the first to use body density as the norm standard in the assessment of body fat in men based on the relationship demonstrated between the two assessment factors. Abdominal, chest, and arm skinfold measures relative to fat and fat-free components were related through developed density–fat measure formulations. Sloan et al.[76] devised a similar formulation for women by assessing abdominal and arm skinfold measurements in reference to body density. Sloan and Weir,[75] utilizing the body density formulations of Brozek et al.,[13] established fat percentage norms for men and women based on thigh and subscapular, and supra-iliac and triceps measurements, respectively, and developed a nomogram for predictive assessment purposes.

Recent developments in this area of study have been directed toward the formulation of generalized equation norms for fat assessment purposes.[2] Generalized equations are drawn from large heterogeneous samples that include a wide range of age levels and are, therefore, more inclusive and applicable to a larger variety of diverse populations.[19,34,35,55] Baun et al.[2] developed a nomogram for the determination of body

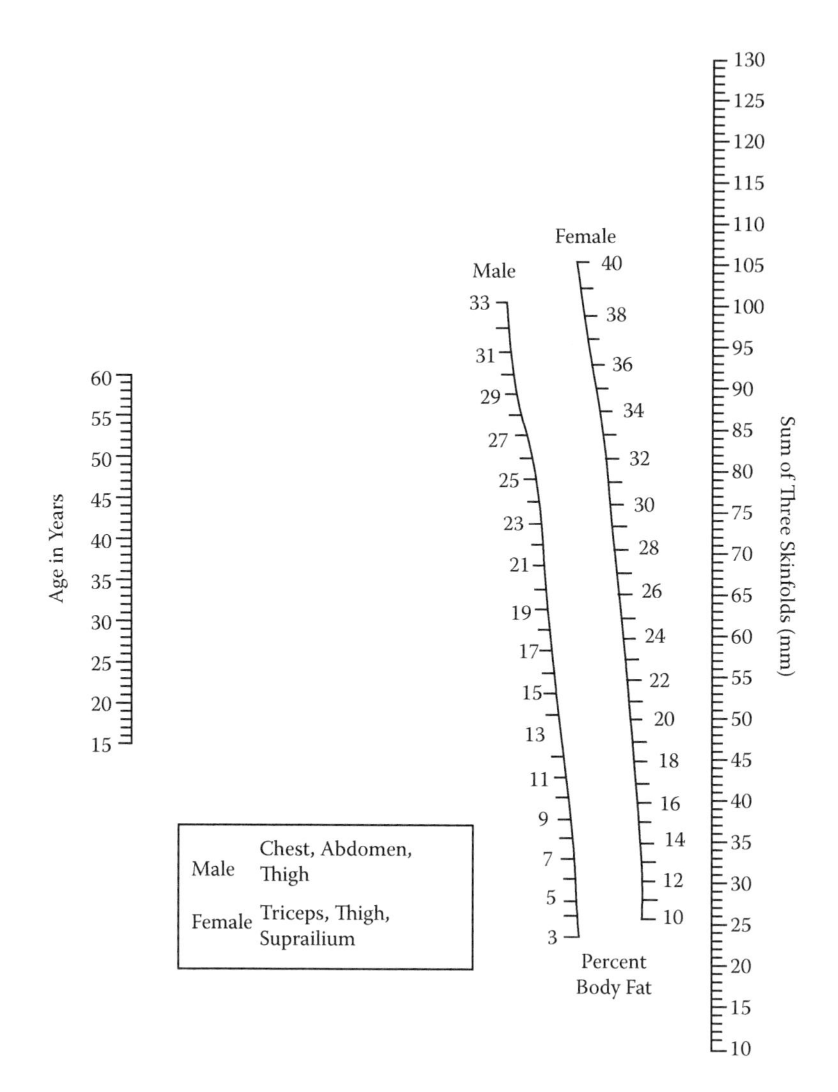

FIGURE 3.3 Nomogram for estimation of body fat. (From Baun, W.B., M.R. Baun, and P.B. Raven, *Research Quarterly for Exercise and Sport,* 52, 380–384, 1981. With the permission of the American Alliance for Health, Physical Education, Recreation, and Dance.)

fat (chest, abdomen, and thigh measurements for men, and triceps, thigh, and iliac crest measurements for women) based on age level and the generalized equations developed by Jackson and Pollack[34] and Jackson et al.[35] (Figure 3.3 and Appendix 3).

Besides skeletal and skinfold evaluations, circumference measurement of specific body sites has also been used in the assessment of fat and fat-free body composition. Wright and Wilmore[94] found that body weight and abdominal circumference measures were significantly related to underwater weighing criteria measures. Similarly, McArdle et al.[52] used a combination of three circumference measurements that were found to be significantly related to body density and fat

TABLE 3.4
Mean Percentage of Body Fat by Sport: Men

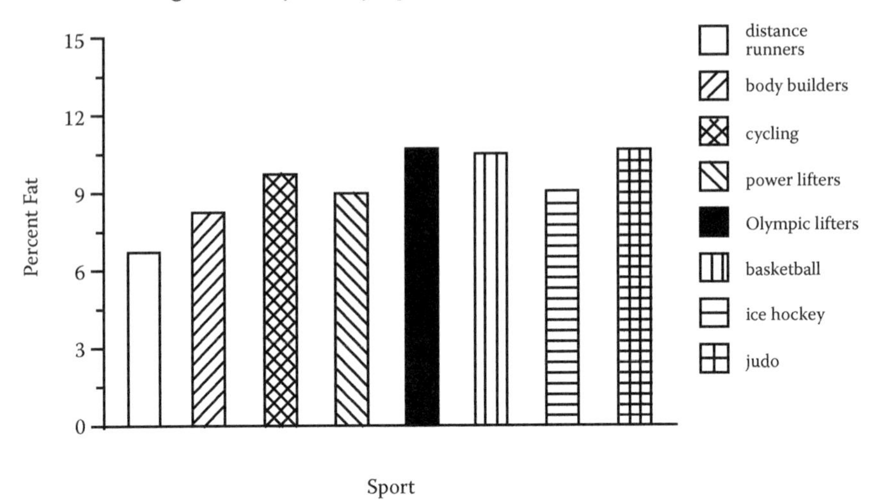

Source: From Slaughter, M.H. and C.B. Christ, in *Body Composition Techniques in Health and Disease.* Davis, R.S.W. and T.J. Cole, Eds., Cambridge University Press, New York, 1995. With permission.

percentage values determined by hydrostatic weighing assessments. Norm constants were developed for the measures taken and utilized in formulas that were age adjusted for younger and older men and women subjects. Wright et al.[95] developed an equation utilizing abdomen and neck circumference measures, and found that it best exemplified percentage of body fat determinations when compared to other anthropometric methods of assessment in field situations in the military. Studies have generally shown that a combination of skinfold and circumference measures would more accurately predict the fat and fat-free components of the body.[46,49,85]

BODY COMPOSITION AND PHYSICAL PERFORMANCE

The relationship of body composition to physical performance has been substantially studied. Within this framework, fat and fat-free assessments have been used to primarily establish norm levels for athletes, to study the effects of lean body and fat body mass on performance, and to investigate the chronic changes of training on performance (Tables 3.4 and 3.5).[8,24,54,79]

In reference to the establishment of norm levels of muscle and fat distribution in athletes, the results of studies have generally shown that:[5,7,8,17,21,24,33,43,52,56,57,64,65,66,69,74,79,82,88,89,91]

1. All of the athletes had less percentage of body fat than did their nonathletic counterparts relative to average established percentage of fat values.

TABLE 3.5
Mean Percentage of Body Fat by Sport: Women

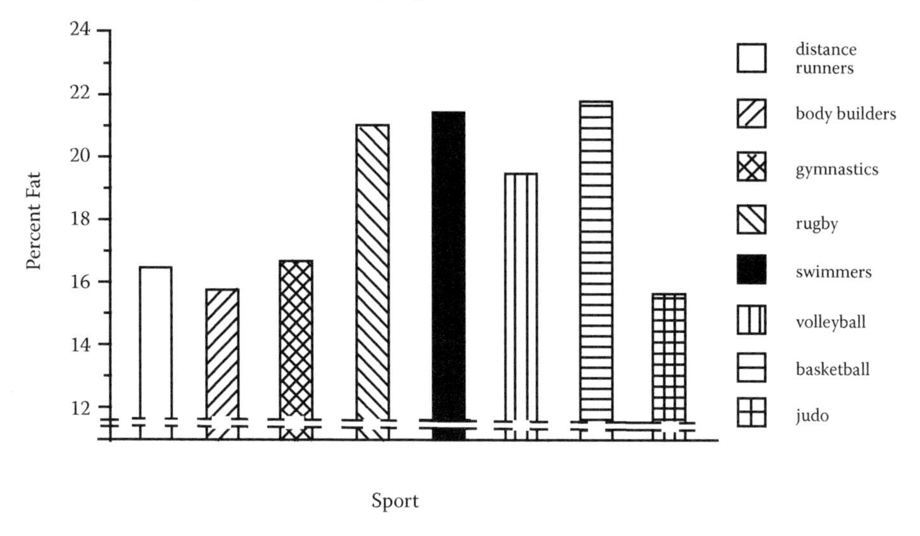

Source: From Slaughter, M.H. and C.B. Christ, in *Body Composition Techniques in Health and Disease.* Davis, R.S.W. and T.J. Cole, Eds., Cambridge University Press, New York, 1995. With permission.

2. Generally, athletes in weight-supported sports (canoeing, kayaking, and swimming) had higher percentages of body fat than did other athletes.
3. The body composition of athletes in the strength and power sports demonstrated higher levels of lean body weight than did those in distance running.
4. Athletes in sports in which competitive participation was determined by weight classes (boxing and wrestling) and those in activities that were anaerobic and aerobic (sprinting and marathon running) had the lowest percentage of body fat among the athletes studied.
5. Athletes in sports in which selective body size was advantageous (basketball, football, volleyball, and rowing) had the highest lean body weights, and those in activities that were aerobic tended to have the lowest lean body weight among the athletes studied.
6. Body fat norms for given sports activities were different for elite male and female athletes.

Studies have shown both positive and negative effects of muscle and fat on performance. Muscle or fat-free tissue generally has a favorable effect on performance, since it is related to the production and conduction of force, whereas excess fat reportedly increases the metabolic cost of exercise.[8,52,57,68,86] Increased amounts of fat-free body mass have been reported to be related to maximum oxygen consumption levels.[22,29,37,60,61,78,93] A lean body mass has also been found to be a favorable predictor of success in weight-supported and strength and power sports.[10,27,52,84] Body fat, however, can be of positive value in contact sports and distance swimming.[18] Too little body fat may result in a decrease in performance effectiveness.

In relation to the chronic effects of training on body composition, studies have reportedly found that compositional changes due to training demonstrated the following:[1,26,41,44,60,62,63,71,76,92]

1. Little or no change in overall weight.
2. Moderate decrease in body fat.
3. Moderate increase in lean body weight.
4. Changes were activity specific and related to level of training.

Pollock and Jackson[58] corroborated these results in an investigation of adult men and women. They found general reductions in body weight and percentage of body fat. Katch and Katch[40] also reported similar results in their study of professional football players. Over a 4-year period, body weight and body fat were both reduced.

SUMMARY

The results of body composition studies relative to physical performance have shown that:

1. Body composition analysis of the fat and lean components of the body can be determined through direct and indirect methods of research.
2. Direct methods employ cadaver studies, whereas indirect measurement methods of investigation incorporate: densitometry, dilution, total body nitrogen, total body potassium content, x-ray, computed tomography, magnetic resonance, ultrasound, electrical conductivity evaluation, infrared interactance, photon absorptiometry, air displacement plethysmography, and anthropmetric measures.
3. The body composition levels of lean body mass and body fat in athletes differ from those of their nonathletic counterparts.
4. In reference to athletes, body composition norm classification guidelines have been established for selected sports activities.
5. Generally, athletes who participate in distance activities have less fat than do those who participate in intense and explosive activities of short duration.
6. Generally, athletes in weight-supported sports have higher percentages of body fat than do other athletes.
7. Athletes in sports in which competitive participation is determined by weight classes and those in activities that are aerobic and anaerobic have the lowest percentage of body fat.
8. Athletes in sports in which selective body size is advantageous have the highest lean body weights.
9. Muscle and fat generally have positive and negative effects on physical activity, respectively.

10. Body composition changes due to physical training include little change in body weight, moderate decrease in body fat, and moderate increase in lean body weight. The compositional changes are activity specific and related to the level of training.

GLOSSARY

Air displacement plethysmography The measure of the air displacement volume of the body to determine the body composition values of fat and fat-free ratios

Anthropometry The measure of fat and fat-free body tissues through the utilization of skeletal, skinfold, and circumference methods of analysis

Body composition The determination and analysis of the fat and lean components of the body

Circumference measurements The measure of body girths from designated body sites

Computed tomography and magnetic resonance imaging The use of x-ray beam and magnetic scanning procedures to produce a cross-sectional image of the fat and fat-free tissues of the body

Densitometric The measure of specific gravity and body density through water volume displacement of weight in air and weight in water

Dilutional (total body water) The use of isotopic deuterium and tritium oxide dilutions to estimate water content and body cellular mass

Dual body photon absorptiometry Two-energy-level photon scans of the body through which the energy differences observed can determine the mineral bone mass of the body

Infrared interactance The use of an electromagnetic radiation body probe to measure the absorptive and reflective spectrographic chemical properties of fat, water, and protein

Neutron activation analysis The measurement of total body nitrogen through gamma ray emissions used to determine the amount of protein in muscle and nonmuscle tissue

Scintillation counter A device that can measure bodily radioactive emissions

Skeletal measures The measure of bone breadths and lengths from designated body sites

Total body electrical conductivity and bioelectric impedance Electromagnetic radiation waves used to measure the electrolyte tissue content and electrical conductivity (reactive/resistance) flow through the body

Total body potassium The gamma-ray measure of the potassium content of the body used to determine the cellular mass of muscle and nonmuscle components

Ultrasound The use of high-frequency sound waves to identify and quantify the density levels of body tissues

X-ray Radiographic analysis of the thickness levels of bone, muscle, and fat

REFERENCES

1. Abernathy, B. et al., *The Biophysical Foundations of Human Movement,* 2nd ed., Human Kinetics, Baltimore, 2005.
2. Baun, W.B., M.R. Baun, and P.B. Raven, A nomogram for the estimate of percent body fat from generalized equations, *Research Quarterly for Exercise and Sport,* 52, 380–384, 1981.
3. Behnke, A.R., Quantitative assessment of body build, *Journal of Applied Physiology,* 16, 960, 1961.
4. Behnke, A.R. and J.H. Wilmore, *Evaluation and Regulation of Body Build and Composition,* Prentice-Hall, Englewood Cliffs, NJ, 1974.
5. Behnke, A.R. and J. Royce, Body size, shape, and composition of several types of athletes, *Journal of Sports Medicine and Physical Fitness,* 6, 75–88, 1966.
6. Behnke, A.R., B.G. Feen, and W.C. Welham, The specific gravity of healthy men: body weight volume as an index of obesity, *Journal of American Medical Association,* 118, 495–498, 1942.
7. Bloomfield, J., R.R. Ackland, and B.C. Elliott, *Applied Anatomy and Biomechanics in Sport,* Blackwell Scientific Publications, Boston, 1994.
8. Boileau, R.A. and C.A. Horswill, Body composition in sports: measurement and applications for weight loss and gain, in *Exercise and Sport Science,* Garrett, W.E. and D.T. Kirkendall, Eds., Lippincott, Williams, and Wilkins, Philadelphia, 2000.
9. Brooks, G.A., T.D. Fahey, and T.P. White, *Exercise Physiology: Human Bioenergetics and Its Application,* 2nd ed., Mayfield Publication Company, Mountain View, CA, 1995.
10. Brown, S.P., W.C. Miller, and J.M. Eason, *Exercise Physiology: Basis of Human Movement in Health and Disease,* Lippincott, Williams, and Wilkins, Baltimore, 2006.
11. Brozek, J., Measuring nutrition, *American Journal of Physical Antropometry,* 11, 147–180, 1953.
12. Brozek, J. and A. Keys, Evaluation of leanness-fatness in man: a survey of methods, *Nutrition Abstracts Review,* 20, 247–256, 1951.
13. Brozek, J., F. Grande, J. Anderson, and A. Keyes, Densitometric analysis of body composition: revision of some quantitative assumptions, *Annals of the New York Academy of Science,* 110, 113–140, 1963.
14. Cerny, F.J. and H.W. Burton, *Exercise Physiology for Health Care Professionals,* Human Kinetics Publishers, Champaign, IL, 2001.
15. Cheline, A.J. The business of body composition, *Fitness Management,* 19, 24–26, September, 2003.
16. Cureton, T.K. *Physical Fitness, Appraisal and Guidance,* Kimpton, Condon, 1947.
17. Dolgner, F.A., T.C. Spasoff, and W.E. St. John, Body build and body composition of high ability female dancers, *Research Quarterly for Exercise and Sport,* 51, 599–607, 1980.
18. Drinkwater, D.T. and J.C. Mazza, Body composition, in *Kinanthropometry in Aquatic Sports: A Study of World Class Athletes,* Carter, J.E.L. and T.R. Ackland, Eds., Human Kinetics Publishers, Champaign, IL, 1994.
19. Durnin, J.V.A. and J. Wormsly, Body fat assessed from total body density and its estimation from skinfold thickness: measurements of 481 men and women ranged from 16–72 years, *British Journal of Nutrition,* 32, 77–97, 1974.
20. Edwards, D.A.W., Observations on the distribution of subcutaneous fat, *Clinical Science,* 9, 305–315, 1950.

21. Fahey, T.D. and C.H. Brown, The effects of anabolic steroids on the strength, body composition, and endurance of college males when accompanied by a weight training program, *Medicine and Science in Sports,* 5, 272–296, 1973.
22. Fahey, T.D., L. Akka, and R. Rolph, Body composition and VO_2 max of exceptional weight-trained athletes, *Journal of Applied Physiology,* 39, 559–561, 1975.
23. Fanelli, M.T. and R.J. Kuczmarski, Ultrasound as an approach to assessing body composition, *American Journal of Clinical Nutrition,* 39, 703–709, 1984.
24. Fleck, S.J., Percentage of body fat of various groups of athletes, *National Strength and Conditionaing Association Journal*, 5, 46–47, 1983.
25. Fox, E., R. Bowers, and M. Foss, *The Physiological Basis for Exercise and Sport,* 5th ed., Brown and Benchmark, Madison, WI, 1993.
26. Gettman, L.R. et al., The effect of circuit weight training on strength, cardiorespiratory function, and body composition of adult men, *Medicine and Science in Sports,* 10, 171–176, 1978.
27. Gettman, L.R., et al., Physiological effects on adult men of circuit strength training and jogging, *Archives of Physical Medicine and Rehabilitation,* 60, 115–120, 1979.
28. Gibson, R.S., *Principles of Nutritional Assessment,* Oxford University Press, New York, 1990.
29. Girandola, R.N., Body composition changes in women: effects of high and low exercise intensity, *Archives of Physical Medicine and Rehabilitation,* 57, 297–300, 1976.
30. Girandola, R.N. and V.L. Katch, Effects of nine weeks of physical training on aerobic capacity and body composition in college men, *Archives of Physical Medicine and Rehabilitation,* 54, 521–524, 1973.
31. Harrison, G.G. and T.B. Van Itallie. Estimation of body composition: a new approach based on electromagnetic principles. *American Journal of Clinical Nutrition,* 35, 1176–1179, 1982.
32. Heyward, V.N., *Advanced Fitness Assessment and Exercise Prescription,* Human Kinetics Publishers, Champaign, IL, 1991.
33. Howley, E.T. and B.D. Franks, *Health Fitness Instructor's Handbook,* 4th ed., Human Kinetics Publishers, Champaign, IL, 2003.
34. Jackson, A.A. and M.L. Pollock, Generalized equations or predicting body density of men, *British Journal of Nutrition,* 40, 497–504, 1978.
35. Jackson, A.A., M.L. Pollock, and A. Ward, Generalized equations for predicting body density of women, *Medicine and Science in Exercise,* 12, 175–182, 1980.
36. Jensen, M.D., Research techniques for body composition assessment, *Journal of the American Dietetic Association,* 92, 454–460, 1992.
37. Johnson, R.E., J.A. Mastropaolo, and M.A. Wharton, Exercise, dietary intake, and body composition, *Journal of the American Dietetic Association,* 61, 399–403, 1972.
38. Katch, F.I. and V.L. Katch, Evaluation of body composition, in *Fitness: Theory and Practice,* 2nd ed., Jordan, P., Ed., Aerobics and Fitness Association of America, Sherman Oaks, CA, 1995.
39. Katch, F.I. and V.L. Katch, *Exercise Physiology: Energy, Nutrition, and Human Performance,* 3rd ed., Lea and Febiger, Philadelphia, 1991.
40. Katch, F.I. and V.L. Katch, The body composition profile: techniques of measurement and applications, *Clinics in Sports Medicine,* 3, 31–63, 1984.
41. Kell, R.T., G. Bell, and A. Quinney, Musculoskeletal fitness, health outcomes, and quality of life, *Sports Medicine,* 31, 863–873, 2001.
42. Keys, A. and J. Brozek, Overweight versus obesity in the evaluation of calorie needs, *Metabolism,* 6, 425, 1957.

43. Lee, H. et al., Physiological characteristics of successful mountain bikers and professional road cyclists, *Journal of Sports Sciences,* 20, 1001–1008, 2002.
44. Lewis, S. et al., Effects of physical activity on weight reduction in obese middle-aged women, *American Journal of Clinical Nutrition,* 29, 151–156, 1976.
45. Lohman, T.G., *Advances in Body Composition Assessment,* Human Kinetics Publishers, Champaign, IL, 1992.
46. Lohman, T.G., Anthropometry and body composition, in *Anthropometric Standardization Reference Manual,* Lohman, T.G., A.E. Roche, and R. Martorell, Eds., Human Kinetics Publishers, Champaign, IL, 1988.
47. Lucaski, H.C. et al., A comparison of body composition including neutron activation analysis of total body nitrogen, *Metabolism,* 30, 777–782, 1981.
48. Lucaski, H.C. et al. Assessment of fat free mass using bioelectric impedance measurements of the human body. *American Journal of Clinical Nutrition,* 41, 810–817, 1985.
49. Malina, R.M., Anthropometry, in *Physiological Assessment of Human Fitness,* Maud, P.J. and C. Foster, Eds., Human Kinetics Publishers, Champaign, IL, 1995.
50. Martin, A.D. and D.T. Drinkwater, Variability in the measure of body fat, *Sports Medicine,* 1, 277–288, 1991.
51. Matiegka, J., The testing of physical efficiency, *American Journal of Physical Anthropology,* 4, 223–230, 1921.
52. McArdle, W.D., F.I. Katch, and V.L. Katch, *Exercise Physiology: Energy, Nutrition, and Human Performance,* 6th ed., Lippincott, Williams, and Wilkins, Philadelphia, 2006.
53. Mendez, J. et al., Total body water by D_20 dilution using saliva samples and gas chromotography, *Journal of Applied Physiology,* 28, 354–357, 1970.
54. National Collegiate Athletic Association, *Sports Medicine Handbook, Assessment of Body Composition,* 15th ed., National Collegiate Athletic Association, Indianapolis, IN, 2002.
55. Nieman, D.C., *Fitness and Sports Medicine: A Health Relatated Approach,* 3rd ed., Bull Publishing Company, Palo Alto, CA, 1995.
56. Noakes, T., *Lore of Running,* 4th ed., Human Kinetics Publishers, Champaign, IL, 2002.
57. Plowman, S.A. and D.L. Smith, *Exercise Physiology for Health Fitness and Performance,* 2nd ed., Benjamin Cummings, San Francisco, 2003.
58. Pollock, M.L. and A.A. Jackson, *Body Composition: Measurement and Changes Resulting from Physical Training, Proceedings of the National College Physical Education Association for Men.* Human Kinetics Publishers, Champaign, IL, 1977.
59. Pollock, M.L., L. Garzarella, and J.E. Graves, The measurement of body composition, in *Physiological Assessment of Human Fitness,* Maud, P.J. and C. Foster, Eds., Human Kinetics Publishers, Champaign, IL, 1995.
60. Pollock, M.L. et al., Effects of walking on body composition and cardiovascular function of middle-aged men, *Journal of Applied Physiology,* 30, 126–130, 1971.
61. Pollock, M.L. et al., Effects of mode training on cardiovascular functions and body composition of adult men, *Medicine and Science in Sports,* 7, 139–145, 1975.
62. Pollock, M.L. et al., Effects of training two days per week at different intensities on middle-aged men, *Medicine and Science in Sports,* 4, 192–197, 1972.
63. Pollock, M.L. et al., Physiologic responses of men 49–65 years of age to endurance training, *Journal of the American Geriatric Society,* 24, 97–104, 1976.
64. Pollock, M.L. et al., Body composition of elite male distance runners, *Annals of the New York Academy of Science,* 301, 361–370, 1977.

65. Pollock, M.L. et al., Body composition of Olympic speed skating candidates, *Research Quarterly for Exercise and Sport,* 53, 150–155, 1982.
66. Powers, S.K. and E.T. Howley, *Exercise Physiology: Theory and Application to Fitness and Performance,* 5th ed., McGraw-Hill, New York, 2004.
67. Presta, E. et al., Comparison in man of total body electrical conductivity and lean body mass derived from body density: validation of a new body composition method, *Metabolism,* 32, 524–527, 1983.
68. Presta, E. et al., Measurement of total body electrical conductivity: a new method for estimation of body composition, *American Journal of Clinical Nutrition,* 37, 735–739, 1983.
69. Raven, P.B. et al., A physiological evaluation of professional soccer players, *British Journal of Sports Medicine,* 10, 209–216, 1976.
70. Robergs, R.A. and S.J. Keteyian, *Fundamentals of Exercise Physiology: for Fitness, Performance, and Health,* 2nd ed., McGraw-Hill, New York, 2003.
71. Russo, E.G. et al., Skinfolds and body composition of sports participants, *The Journal of Sports Medicine and Physical Fitness,* 32, 303–313, September, 1992.
72. Schulz, L.O. and C.F. Douthitt, Bioelectrical impedance analysis, A research tool useful for classroom teaching, *Journal of Nutrition Education,* 22, 182D, 1990.
73. Siri, W.E., Body composition from fluid spaces and density, in *Techniques for Measuring Body Composition,* Brozek, J. and A. Henschel, Eds., National Academy of Sciences National Research Council, Washington, DC, pp. 223–244, 1961.
74. Slaughter, M.H. and T.G. Lohman, An objective method for measurement of musculoskeletal size to characterize body physique with application to the athletic population, *Medicine and Science in Sports and Exercise,* 12, 170–174, 1980.
75. Sloan, A.W. and J.J. Weir, Nomograms for prediction of body density and total body fat from skinfold measurements, *Journal of Applied Physiology,* 28, 221–222, 1970.
76. Sloan, A.W., J.J. Burt, and C.S. Blyth, Estimation of body fat in young women, *Journal of Applied Physiology,* 17, 967, 1967.
77. Smith, D.P. and F.W. Stransky, The effect of training and detraining on the body composition and cardiovascular response of young women to exercise, *Journal of Sports Medicine,* 16, 112–120, 1976.
78. Spenst, L.F., A.D. Martin, and D.T. Drinkwater, Muscle mass of competitive male athletes, *Journal of Sports Sciences,* 11, 3–8, 1993.
79. Sprynarova, S. and J. Parzkova, Functional capacity and body composition in top weight-lifters, swimmers, runners, and skiers, *Internationale Zeitschrift fur Angewandte Physiologie Einschliesslich Arbeitsphysiologie,* 29, 184–194, 1971.
80. Van Dobeln, W., Fat free body weight of Swedish Air Force pilots, *Aerospace Medicine,* 32, 67–69, 1961.
81. Wagner, D.R. and V.H. Heyward, Techniques of body composition assessment: a review of laboratory and field methods, *Research Quarterly for Exercise and Sport,* 70, 135, 1999.
82. Welham, W.C. and A.R. Behnke, The specific graffiti of healthy men, *Journal of the American Medical Association,* 118, 498, 1942.
83. Wildman, R.E.C. and B.S. Miller, *Sports and Fitness Nutrition,* Wadsworth, Thomson Learning, Belmont, CA, 2004.
84. Wilmore, J.H., Alterations in strength, body composition and anthropometric measurements consequent to a 10-week weight training program, *Medicine and Science in Sports,* 6, 133–138, 1974.
85. Wilmore, J.H., Body composition in sports and exercise: directions for future research, *Medicine and Science in Sports and Exercise,* 15, 21–31, 1983.

86. Wilmore, J.H. Sports medicine, in *Anthropometric Standardization Reference Manual,* Lohman, T.G., A.E. Roche, and R. Mortorell, Eds., Human Kinetics Publishers, Champaign, IL, 1988.
87. Wilmore, J.H. and A.R. Behnke, Predictability of lean body weight through anthropometric assessment in college men, *Journal of Applied Physiology,* 25, 349, 1968.
88. Wilmore, J.H. and D.L. Costill, *Physiology of Sport and Exercise,* 3rd ed., Human Kinetics Publishers, Champaign, IL, 2004.
89. Wilmore, J.H. and W. Haskell, Body composition and endurance capacity of professional football players, *Journal of Applied Physiology,* 33, 564–567, 1972.
90. Wilmore, J.H., J. Royce, R.N. Girandola, F.I. Katch, and V.L. Katch, Body composition changes with a 10-week program of jogging, *Medicine and Science in Sports,* 2, 113–117, 1970.
91. Wilmore, J.H., C.H. Brown, and J.A. Davis, Body physique and composition of the female distance runner, *Annals of the New York Academy of Science,* 301, 764–776, 1977.
92. Wilmore, J.H. et al., Physiological alterations consequent to circuit weight training, *Medicine and Science in Sports,* 10, 79–84, 1978.
93. Wilmore, J.H. et al., Physiological alterations consequent to 20-week conditioning programs of bicycling, tennis, and jogging, *Medicine and Science in Sports and Exercise,* 12, 1–8, 1980.
94. Wright, H.F. and J.H. Wilmore, Estimation of relative body fat and lean body weight in a United States Marine Corps population, *Aerospace Medicine,* 45, 301–306, 1974.
95. Wright, H.F., C.O. Dotson, and P.O. Davis, A simple technique for measurement of percent fat in man, *U.S. Navy Medicine,* 72, 23–27, 1981.

Part Two

Physical and Physiological Conditioning

4 Muscular Strength and Muscular Endurance

INTRODUCTION

The development of muscular strength and muscular endurance through physical training is significant to overall muscle fitness and function in performance. Muscular strength can be defined as the maximal exertion of force against resistance, whereas muscular endurance can be described as the submaximal repetitive or sustained exertion of force against resistance. Both components are developed during conditioning processes in an interrelated manner relative to the number of repetitions and the load lifted.

MUSCLE STRUCTURE AND MUSCLE CONTRACTION

Skeletal muscle is basically composed of muscle fibers and myofibrils. The muscle fibers or cells are individually enclosed in layers of endomysium connective tissue, bound together in bundles of fasciculi, and covered by perimysium tissue. Muscle fasciculi are then combined to form specific muscle tissue and are held together by epimysium and fascia band coverings, respectively (Figure 4.1).

Muscle fibers contain cytoplasm or sarcoplasm within which are found mitochondria and myofibrils covered by a plasma membrane or sarcolemma. A membranous system of channels made up of sarcoplasmic reticuli or storage areas and transverse tubules or pathways, cross through the cellular sarcoplasm. The myofibrils are composed of actin and myosin, light and dark protein filaments. These filaments are arranged in units of sarcomeres bound by Z lines surrounding I and A, light and dark band filament sections. During muscle contraction, the Z-lined sections move toward the center and shorten, the I bands narrow, and the A bands remain the same, relative to length (Figure 4.2).[4]

Muscle contraction processes begin with the release of acetylcholine from the motor end plate of a motor neuron due to electrical and chemical stimulus depolarization (Figure 4.3).[39] In turn, muscle cell membrane depolarization occurs, and the acetylcholine is conducted through the transverse tubules, generating action potential impulses throughout the fibers innervated. Calcium ions are then secreted from the sarcoplasmic reticulum and attach themselves to the tropomyosin–troponin complex (protein process governing substances).[25] This process results in a conformational change in the position of actin, allowing the myosin globular heads to bind to these sites (Figure 4.4). These globular heads contain myosin adenosine triphos-

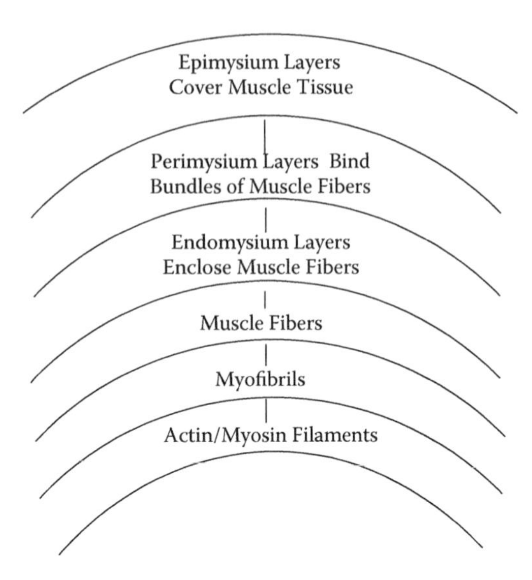

FIGURE 4.1 Muscle structure.

phatase (ATPase) enzymes which are activated upon binding. At this point, adenosine triphosphate (ATP) splits and energy is released. Muscle contraction occurs when the myosin globular arms or heads pull the actin filaments toward the center in a ratchet action.

MUSCLE FIBER TYPES

There are basically two muscle fiber types, slow twitch and fast twitch. Twitch refers to contraction response to stimuli. Type I (slow oxidative) fibers are high in aerobic capacity, slow in contraction speed, high in fatigue resistance, and low in force production. Type II A and Type II B fibers, two fast-twitch subtypes (fast oxidative/glycolytic and fast glycolytic), are high in anaerobic capacity, fast in contraction speed, low in fatigue resistance, and high in force production. In reference to resistance training, slow-twitch fibers, because of their low force production, would be used for low-to-moderate-resistance, high-repetitive muscle endurance activities, whereas fast-twitch fibers, because of their high force production, would be used for high-resistance, low-repetitive muscle strength activities (Figure 4.5).[22]

MUSCLE STRENGTH AND MUSCLE ENDURANCE DETERMINANTS

Muscular strength and muscular endurance development can basically be determined by muscle size and cross section, muscle length and angle of pull, and muscle contraction speed and force production. There is a significant relationship between muscle size and cross section, and the generation of muscle strength.[3,19] The larger the size and cross section, the greater the force produced. This relationship is

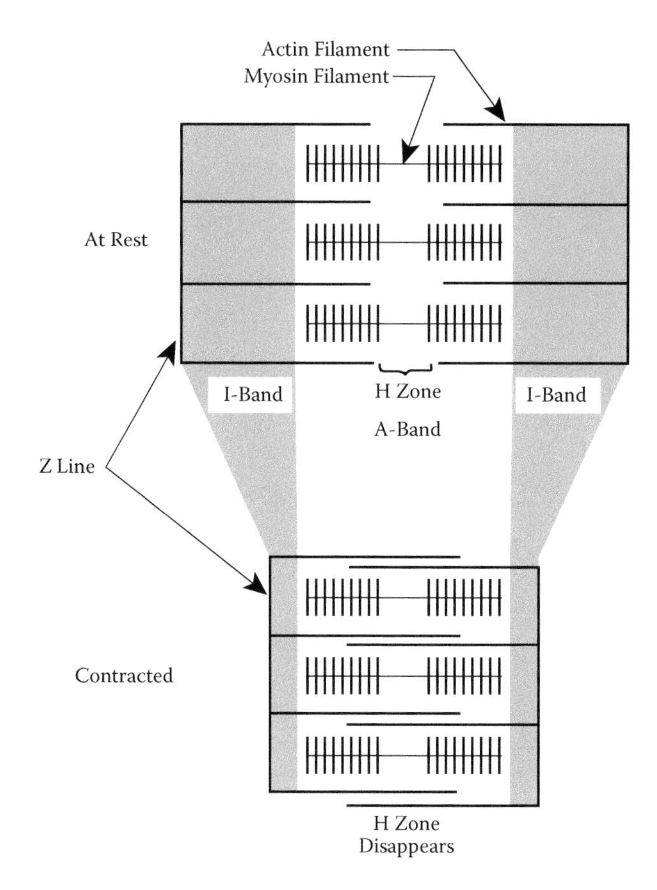

FIGURE 4.2 Muscular contraction mechanics. The interaction of the actin-myosin filaments in the contraction of skeletal muscle. (From Bowers, R.W. and E.L. Fox, *Sport Physiology,* 3rd ed., W.C. Brown Publishers, Dubuque, IA, 1992. Reproduced with the permission of the McGraw-Hill Companies.)

attributed to the hypertrophy of the myofibrils in size and number, which activates a greater amount of actin–myosin cross bridges.[14,17,26,32,34,42]

Force production can be shown as an interaction between muscle length and angle of pull. While the greatest force production occurs with muscle tissue at extended length, the greatest force production relative to angle of pull is set at a range of 80° to 120°.[17,29,35] The equal interaction of, or predominance of either length or angle of pull in training must be determined by the type of activity or movement pattern to be executed. The magnitude of actin–myosin cross bridge activation would be the predominant factor, because the production of force would be related to the increasing or decreasing site numbers activated during shortening and lengthening patterns of movement (Figure 4.6).[21–22,29,39]

Muscle contraction speed and force production are based on resistance load.[5,13] As resistance increases, muscle contraction speed slows. Similarly, as resistance decreases, muscle contraction speed increases. The variance in load is the principal

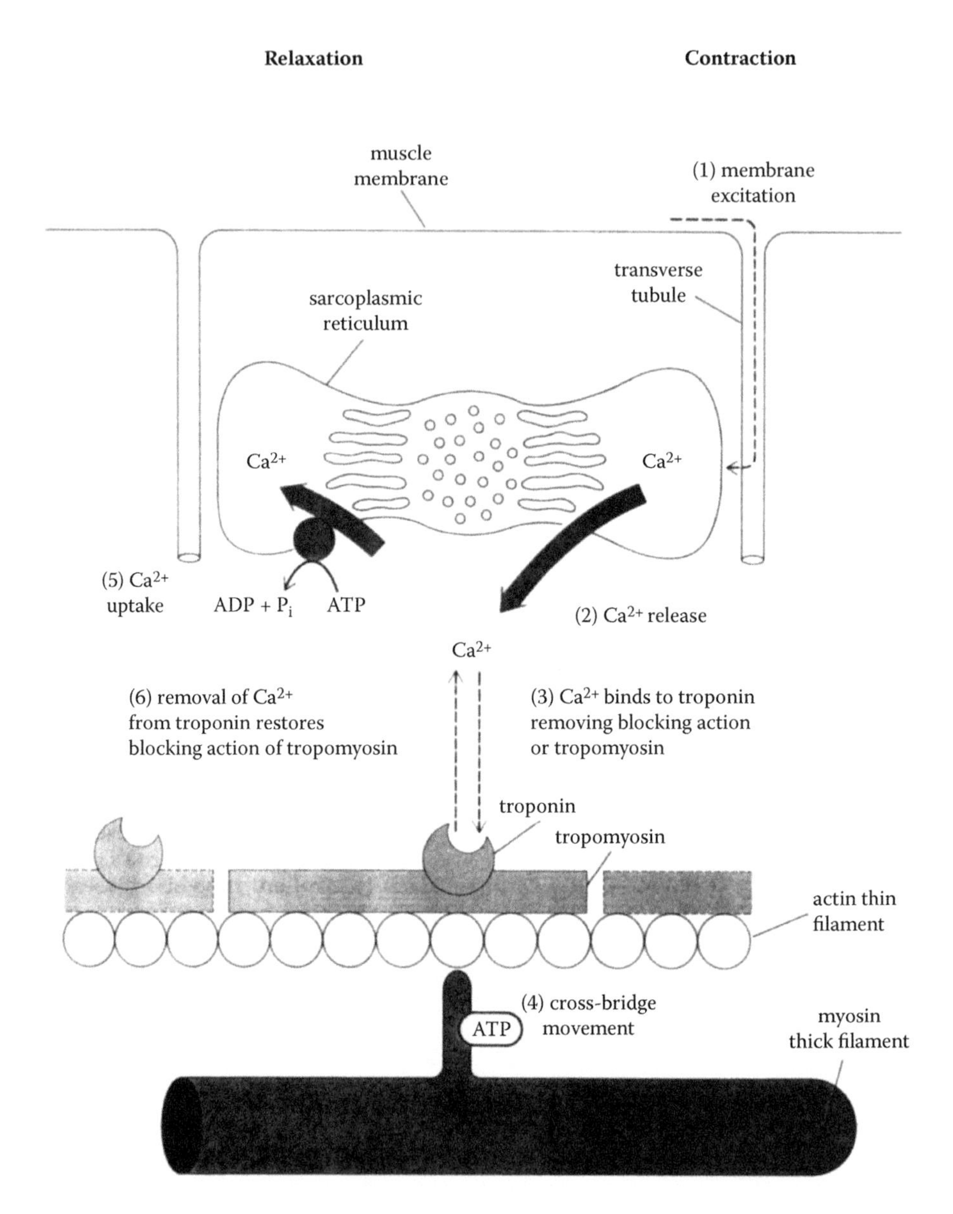

FIGURE 4.3 Diagram of neural excitation and muscle contraction. (From Vander, A.J., J.H. Sherman, and D.S. Luciano, *Human Physiology: The Mechanisms of Body Function,* 3rd ed., McGraw-Hill, New York, 1980. Reproduced with the permission of the McGraw-Hill Companies.)

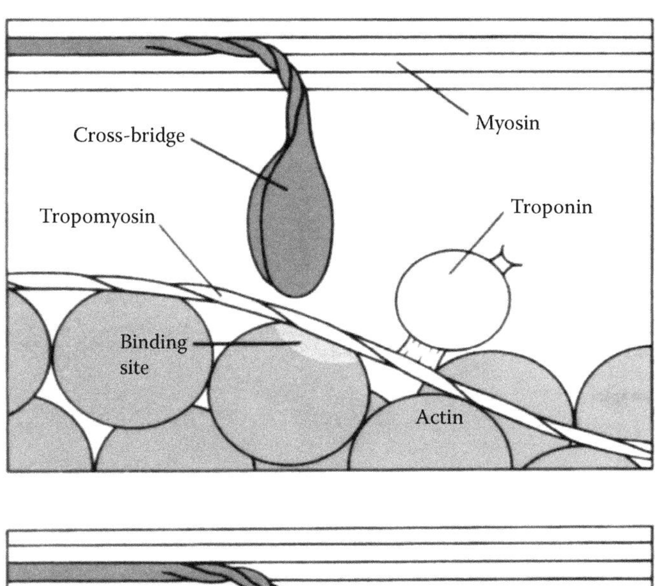

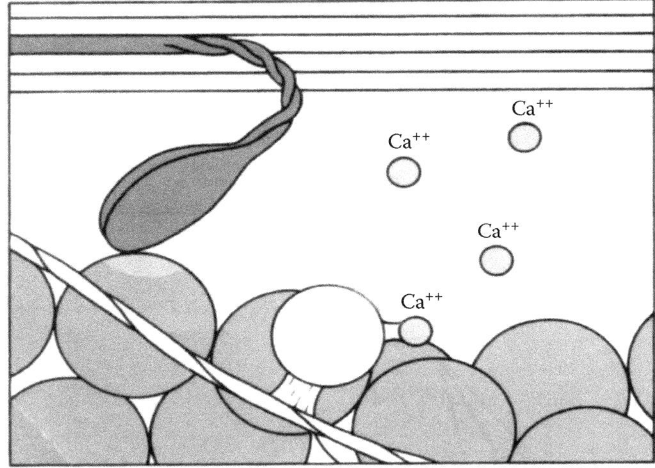

FIGURE 4.4 Calcium ions and muscle contraction. Calcium attachment to troponin and the tropomyosin complex results in a conformational change of the actin filament, exposing the binding sites. Myosin cross bridges can then bind to these sites, and contraction can take place. (From Fox, S.I., *Human Physiology,* 3rd ed., W.C. Brown Publishers, Dubuque, IA, 1990. Reproduced with the permission of the McGraw-Hill Companies.)

MUSCLE STRENGTH TRAINING

Resistance - High

Repetitions - Low

MUSCLE ENDURANCE TRAINING

Resistance - Low to Medium

Repetitions - High

FIGURE 4.5 Weight training. Resistance–repetitions specificity for muscle strength and muscle endurance training.

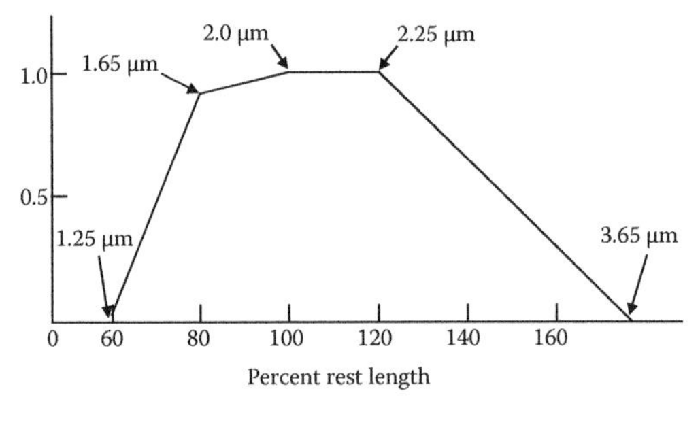

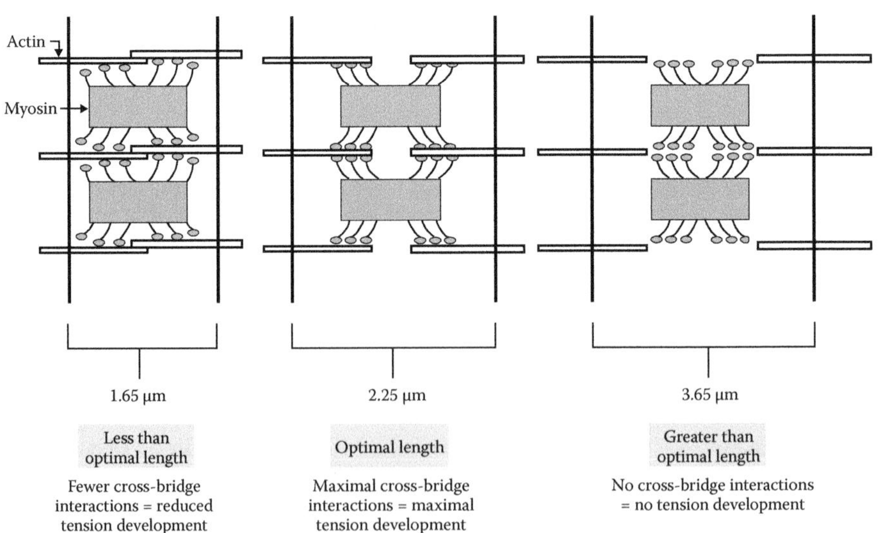

FIGURE 4.6 Length–force relationships of skeletal muscle. (From Powers, S.K. and E.T. Howley, *Exercise Physiology: Theory and Application to Fitness and Performance,* 2nd ed., Brown and Benchmark, Madison, WI, 1994. With permission from The McGraw-Hill Companies.)

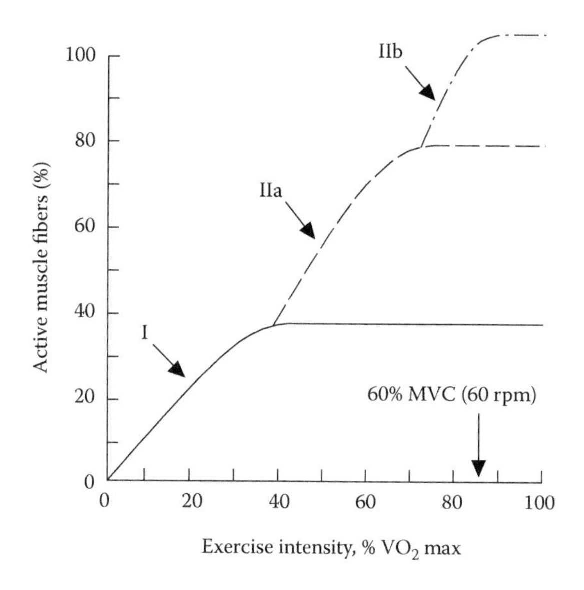

FIGURE 4.7 Muscle fiber recruitment processes relative to increasing intensity. (From Powers S.K. and E.T. Howley, *Exercise Physiology: Theory and Application to Fitness and Performance,* 2nd ed., Brown and Benchmark, Madison, WI, 1994. With permission from The McGraw-Hill Companies.)

factor.[17] Force and speed are accommodative. The complete activation of the actin–myosin cross bridges must be augmented progressively to produce greater force.[22] The time taken for cross bridge activation would affect the speed of the muscle contraction shortening process.[13,40] Slow-twitch muscle fibers contract first; then in turn the fast-twitch fibers sequentially contract relative to increasing intensity (Figure 4.7).[35] Greater training use of fast-twitch muscle fibers in this regard could be significant to the faster and greater production of force.[22,31]

STRENGTH TRAINING PRINCIPLES AND PRACTICES

The development of muscle strength and muscle endurance can be demonstrated through the application of the prevalent strength training principles and practices of progressive resistance, overload, arrangement of exercises, periodization, volume, quantitative and qualitative relationships, and the generality and/or specificity of the training programs implemented.

Progressive resistance and overload practices have become significant applicative factors to the development of muscular strength and muscular endurance. In reference to progressive resistance, muscle tissue must be stressed beyond the normal workload in order to affect motor unit recruitment, size, hypertrophy, and subsequently a development in muscle strength.[25] In this manner, muscle groups generally adapt to the increased workload and the establishment of subsequent greater strength baseline levels. When the predetermined strength goals are reached, maintenance programs are implemented in order to retain the strength gains that have been made.[10]

Total Body Workout:

1. Large before small muscle group exercises
2. Multiple-joint before single-joint exercises
3. Rotation of upper and lower body exercises or opposing (agonist-antagonist relationship) exercises

Upper and Lower Body Split Workout:

1. Large before small muscle group exercises
2. Multiple-joint before single-joint exercises
3. Rotation of opposing exercises (agonist-antagonist relationship)

Muscle Group Split Routines:

1. Multiple-joint before single-joint exercises
2. Higher intensity before lower intensity exercises

FIGURE 4.8 Strength training general exercise sequence order. (From Kraemer, W.J. and N.A. Ratamess, Progression and resistance training, *Research Digest,* President' Council on Physical Fitness, Series 6, No. 3, September, 2005.)

The principle of overload can similarly be initiated through our increase in resistance, number of repetitions, and time utilization. Increased amounts of resistance will produce a muscular overload. High resistance and low numbers of repetitions would be advocated for strength gains.[8,25] The development of muscular endurance is effected through the use of less resistance and increased number of repetitions. In reference to time utilization, slowness of exercise execution relative to designated movement patterns would also increase the generation of muscle force.[41]

The arrangement of exercise order is related to the procedural sequencing of designated priority (Figure 4.8). The upper legs and hip muscles can be exercised first, followed by exercises for the chest and upper arm, back and posterior muscles of the legs, lower legs and ankles, shoulders and posterior muscles of the upper arms, abdomen, and anterior muscles of upper arms.[4] The structural utilization of this exercise order includes total body, upper and lower body, and designated muscle group development programs.[25]

The concepts of periodization and volume may be used in program development.[36,43] Periodization refers to the variability of exercise training programs.[25,30] Different training methodologies related to type, amount, and intensity can be utilized in order to optimize the strength and endurance gains sought throughout varied periods of time schedules. Generally, the variational cycles include an incorporation of hypertrophy, strength, power, peaking, and rest periods of training.[4] The amount and intensity of work are also related to training volume. The manipulation of set and repetition numbers relative to intensity are demonstrative examples. High-volume training refers to low-to-moderate resistance exercises for muscle endurance, whereas low-volume training is related to high-intensive resistance exercises for muscle strength[25]

The production of muscular force can also be determined by the quantitative and qualitative related training processes.[8] Quantitatively, muscle strength gains are the result of increases in the size of muscle fibers and training volume, while qualitative measurements may be assessed by the strength per unit of physiological cross section. In this regard, de Vries[8] reported significant correlations between size and strength in a study of elbow flexion in trained men. Quantitative and qualitative force production can also be the result of motor unit recruitment and rate of innervation.[18,25] Stimulation rate increase in muscle fibers increases the generation of strength in those fibers.

The generality and specificity of muscle force production is influenced by the relationship of muscle groups and muscle function relative to strength training, respectively. While de Vries[8] reported the general relationship among muscle groups to be significant relative to strength, Sale and MacDougall[38] found muscle function to be specific. In a review of related studies, McArdle et al.[32] reported on the generality of strength training. They found nonsignificant differences between two groups trained and tested isotonically and isokinetically, and concentrically and eccentrically, respectively. The predominance of research, however, has demonstrated the evident specificity in strength training.[32,38] Sale and MacDougall[38] found specificity to be related to the muscle fiber type used, the speed of muscular contraction, the amount of force produced, and the designated pattern of movement utilized. The results of such studies indicate that strength training can be of value generally in the development of overall body strength and endurance, which in turn may contribute to success in activities of a physical nature. In relation to the specificity of training, strength programs must be related to purpose, method, and the given parameters of movement.[38]

MUSCULAR STRENGTH AND MUSCULAR ENDURANCE TRAINING PROGRAMS

There are three basic exercise training programs for the development of muscle strength and muscle endurance. They include isotonic, isometric, and isokinetic methods of conditioning (Table 4.1). Isotonic exercises are based on a full range of movement against a constant resistance, and entail the contraction and relaxation of muscle tissue during concentric and eccentric phases of activity. Isometric exercises are based on the contraction of muscle tissue over a short period of time (6 to 8 sec) against an immovable resistance while one maintains a static body position. Isoki-

TABLE 4.1
Isotonic, Isokinetic, and Isometric Resistance Exercises

Resistance Exercises	Movement Pattern	Force/Resistance
Isotonic	Dynamic (Concentric/Eccentric)	Force: Varied/ Resistance: Fixed
Isokinetic	Dynamic (Concentric/Eccentric)	Force: Speed Fixed/ Resistance: Accomodative
Isometric	Static (No Movement)	Force: Fixed/ Resistance: Fixed

netic exercises incorporate maximal muscle contraction over a full range of movement against a variable resistance and are governed by fixed-speed control.

Isotonic resistance training, utilizing free weights or designated resistance equipment, incorporates progressive loads, sets, and repetitions in the development of muscle strength and muscle endurance. Heavy resistance and low numbers of repetitions done within a three-set context would be indicative of a strength development predominance, whereas light to moderate resistance and high numbers of repetitions would be indicative of an endurance development emphasis. Berger[3] advocated six to eight repetitions maximum, three sets per workout, and three to four workouts per week for strength development. DeLorme and Watkins[7] established a program that entailed ten repetitions maximum in ascending resistance order (50, 75, and 100%), three sets per workout, and four workouts per week. Research in this area has shown that six repetitions maximum and three sets have produced greater increases in strength, whereas incremental numbers of repetitions with low-weight resistance have resulted in greater increases in muscle endurance.[1,2,19]

Isometric training usually requires maximal efforts over short periods of time, against an immovable resistance without bodily movement, for the development of muscle strength. Strength gains are specific to the joint angle used for the given exercise, and contraction bouts must be repeated over various joint angles for strength results to become generalized. Such exercises vary in number of bouts, number of seconds that muscle contractions are held, and joint angles used. Sessions are short in time and can be repeated to maximize strength and endurance development. Stationary body positions relative to joint angles and exercises are similar to dynamic isotonic exercise positions. Conditioning routines are also similar in regard to overall large muscle utilization patterns.

Isokinetic training programs incorporate maximal muscular tension and contraction throughout a full range of movement, within set speed controls, for the development of muscle strength and muscle endurance. This type of training is similar to isotonic exercise in terms of nature and scope, but differs in terms of bout length and bout speed. Special hydraulic equipment is necessary for this form of training. Isokinetic research has shown that maximal strength and endurance gains are made specifically at speeds of movement equal to or slower than the established training velocity.[16,27] Training at high-velocity rates results in high-velocity strength and endurance development, while training at low-velocity rates results in low-velocity strength gains.[38]

Comparisons of these three systems of training generally show that isokinetic training produces the greatest muscle strength and muscle endurance rates of development, can be more adaptable to specific movement patterns, promotes less muscle soreness and injury incidence possibilities, and can also contribute to skill improvement.[19,41] Isokinetic methods of training must therefore be considered better than isotonic and isometric approaches to conditioning of this kind. However, because of isokinetic equipment expense and isometric injury possibilities, isotonic methods of conditioning may be the most practical of the three. Isotonic resistance exercises can be done with or without equipment, can offer more than adequate training routines, and can provide effective measures of both strength and endurance.

FLEXIBILITY

Flexibility refers to the extent to which a muscle or group of muscles can functionally move through a range of motion around a joint axis. The movement degree of flexibility is specific to each joint, and is generally limited by joint structure, movement dimension capacity, and the elasticity and extensibility of muscle and connective tissue.[6,41] Flexibility can be separated into static and dynamic components. Fleishman[12] defined static flexibility as the ability to stretch the body in different directions, and dynamic flexibility as the ability to make continuous trunk and limb movements. Although both components refer to range of motion, static flexibility is passive, and dynamic flexibility is movement oriented. Static flexibility can be improved through slow stretching exercises, while dynamic flexibility is enhanced by slow types of muscle contracted movements.[11,33] Both types of flexibility include interaction of muscle spindles and Golgi tendon organs, which govern the amount of stretch involved in the shortening and lengthening of muscle tissue during movement.[35] Muscle spindles facilitate contraction and stretch, while Golgi tendon organs inhibit contraction and stretch to protect muscle tissue from possible injury. Agonistic and antagonistic muscle group synchronization would also be a factor in range movement capacity.[20]

EFFECTS OF RESISTANCE TRAINING PROGRAMS

Resistance training programs bring about a variety of chronic changes in the body relative to muscle and neuromuscular function, muscle size, biochemical adaptations, joint movement capacity, and body composition (Table 4.2).[11,15,20,24]

In reference to muscle function, strength and endurance levels are both increased. Strength rises slowly in the beginning periods of exercise, then builds rapidly for some time, and reaches a plateau or slow rate of gain over the remainder of the program time.[26] Neuromuscular function has been studied through electromyographic analysis; studies have shown that heavy resistance training results in an increase in synchronous electrical patterns with firing of high-threshold motor units, while light resistance training results in an increase in synchronous electrical patterns and firing of low-threshold motor units.[25] There is also an increase in type I and type II muscle fiber cross-sectional diameters as a result of the formation of additional myofibril actin–myosin filaments in response to heavy work.[24,37]

Biochemical changes are also evident in response to training. Increased adenosine triphosphate–phosphocreatine concentrations, decreased mitochondrial density, and decreased aerobic enzyme activity have been reported.[8,11,15,17] In regard to glycolytic enzyme activity, no change due to resistance training has been generally evident.[12,15]

In reference to flexibility, little evidence has been found relative to strength increase, injury reduction, and gain in physical performance.[33] The relationship is more theoretical than evidential[23] Study results have not been significantly definitive relative to increased muscle and joint movement capacities.[23] Research has been centered in static and dynamic investigations. Structural factors that may affect flexibility during training include muscle, tendon, ligament, and bone extensibility.[33]

TABLE 4.2
The Effects of Strength Training on Health and Fitness Variables

Variable	Resistance Exercise
Bone Mineral Density	↑↑
Body Composition	
% fat	↓
LBM	↑↑
Strength	↑↑↑
Glucose Metabolism	
Insulin response to glucose challenge	↓↓
Basal insulin levels	↓
Insulin Sensitivity	↑↑
Serum lipids	
HDL	↑↔
LDL	↓↔
Resting heart rate	↔
Stroke volume	↔
Blood Pressure at rest	
Systolic	↔
Diastolic	↓↔
VO_2 max	↑
Endurance Time	↑↑
Physical function	↑↑↑
Basal metabolism	↑↑

Source: Adapted from Pollock, M.L. and K.R. Vincent, Resistance Training for Health, The President's Council on Physical Fitness and Sports Research Digest, Series 2, No. 8, December, 1996.

Body composition changes due to resistance training include decreased body fat and increased fat-free weight levels.[11,24] The decrease in body fat is related to total energy expenditure relative to the intensity and duration of the exercise program, while fat-free weight increase is related to the heavy resistance nature of the exercise program and the corresponding hypertrophy of muscle tissue.

SUMMARY

Research studies in the area of muscular strength and muscular endurance have demonstrated the following results:

1. The development of muscular strength and muscular endurance is significant to overall muscle fitness and function in performance.
2. The factors that influence strength and endurance development are basically muscle size and cross section, muscle length and angle of pull, and muscle contraction speed and force production.

3. The development of muscle strength and muscle endurance can be demonstrated through the application of the prevalent strength training principles and practices of progressive resistance, overload, arrangement of exercises, quantitative and qualitative muscle relationships, and the generality and specificity of the training programs implemented.
4. Isotonic, isometric, and isokinetic methods of conditioning are used as basic training programs for the development of muscle strength and muscle endurance.
5. The movement degree of flexibility is specific to each joint and is generally limited by joint structure, movement dimension capacity, and the elasticity and extensibility of muscle and connective tissue.
6. Resistance training programs bring about a variety of chronic changes in the body relating to muscle and neuromuscular function, muscle size, biochemical adaptations, joint movement capacity, and body composition.

GLOSSARY

Acetylcholine Chemical substance involved in neural impulse transmission

Actin Thin protein filament found in myofibrils that interacts with myosin in muscle contraction processes

Action potential The electrical activity generated in the process of depolarization in nerve and muscle tissue

Adenosine diphosphate Chemical compound that interacts with inorganic phosphate to form adenosine triphosphate

Adenosine triphosphatase Protein enzyme catalyst involved in muscle contraction processes

Adenosine triphosphate–phosphocreatine Immediate energy compound sources involved in muscle contraction processes

Aerobic enzyme activity Slow-twitch muscle fibers that provide aerobic (oxidative) catalyst activity

Agonist/antagonist Muscle or muscle group that works in concert with one opposite muscle or muscle group in the contraction/relaxation synchronization process during exercise execution

Arrangement of exercises The process in weight training wherein large muscle groups are exercised before the smaller muscle groups

Body composition The fat and fat-free weight of the body

Concentric movement The shortening phase of muscle contraction during isotonic exercise

Cytoplasm/sarcoplasm Cellular fluid

Dynamic flexibility Active and continued muscular movement of the trunk and limbs

Eccentric movement The lengthening phase of muscle contraction during isotonic exercise

Electromyographic analysis The electrical pattern that is demonstrative of muscular function in the firing of motor units

Endomysium Connective tissue layer that covers muscle fibers
Epimysium Layer that covers muscle tissue
Fast-twitch muscle fiber types Muscle fibers that are anaerobic, fast contracting, high in force production, and fast fatiguing
Flexibility The extent to which a muscle or group of muscles can functionally move through a range of motion around a joint axis
Glycolytic enzyme activity Fast-twitch muscle fibers that provide anaerobic (glycolytic) catalyst activity
Golgi tendon organ Sensory receptor that governs the stretching limits of muscle contraction
Hypertrophy An increase in muscle size in response to resistance exercise adaption
Isokinetic exercise Exercise that is executed at a constant speed throughout a full range of movement against an equal designated resistance
Isometric exercise Exercise that is nonmoving, at given body angles, for short periods of time against an immovable resistance
Isotonic exercise Exercise that is based on a full range of movement against a designated and moveable resistance
Mitochondria Energy-producing cellular organelles
Motor end plate Synaptic junction between nerve and muscle tissue
Motor unit The neuron and the innervated muscle fibers involved in muscle contraction processes
Muscle fasciculi Bundles of muscle fibers
Muscle length Determines the contraction generation of muscular force relative to resting, shortening, or lengthening movement patterns
Muscle spindles Intrafusal muscle fibers that are involved in the rate and amount of muscle stretch
Muscle cross section Measure of the diameter of muscle tissue
Muscular endurance Submaximal repetitive or sustained exertion of force against resistance
Muscle size Measure of the magnitude of muscular tissue
Muscular strength Maximal exertion of force against resistance
Myofibrils Contractile components of muscle tissue that contain actin and myosin filaments that are involved in the process of muscle contraction
Myosin Thick protein filament found in myofibrils that interacts with actin in muscle contraction processes
Overload principle An increase in exercise resistance that can be employed through the addition of weight, number of repetitions, or time, over and above the designated norm
Perimysium tissue Connective tissue layer that binds muscles of fibers into bundles
Periodization Refers to the use of variability methodology in resistance training programs
Progressive resistance The periodic increase in weight resistance during the course of a program aimed at muscular strength gain
Repetition maximum The maximum weight lifted in one trial effort
Sarcolemma Membranous muscle tissue that covers individual muscle fibers
Sarcomere Contractile unit of muscle tissue

Sarcoplasmic reticulum Calcium ion storage areas
Slow-twitch muscle fiber types Muscle fibers that are aerobic, slow contracting, low in force production, and slow fatiguing
Specificity The development of strength through designated resistance movement patterns
Static flexibility The stretching and lengthening of muscle tissue to a maximum point
Training volume Low-volume training refers to high-intensity exercises for muscle hypertrophy, whereas high-volume training is related to low-to-moderate exercises for muscle endurance
Transverse tubules Pathways through which neural impulse is conducted in order to activate calcium ions stored in sarcoplasmic reticulum
Tropomyosin–troponin complex Protein process governing substances involved in the contraction of muscle tissue
Z-lines Separate sarcolemma units

REFERENCES

1. Abernathy, B. et al., *The biophysical Foundations of Human Movement,* 2nd ed., Human Kinetics, Baltimore, 2005.
2. American College of Sports Medicine, Position stand: progression models in resistance training for healthy adults, *Medicine and Science in Sports and Exercise,* 34, 364–380, 2002.
3. Berger, R.A., Optimum repetitions for the development of strength. *Research Quarterly,* 33, 334–338, 1962.
4. Brown, S.P., W.C. Miller, and J.M. Eason, *Exercise Physiology: Basis of Human Movement in Health and Disease,* Lippincott, Williams, and Wilkins, Baltimore, 2006.
5. Cerny, F.J. and H.W. Burton, *Exercise Physiology for Health Care Professionals,* Human Kinetics, Champaign, IL, 2001.
6. Corbin, C.B., and R. Lindsey, *Fitness for Life,* 4th ed., Human Kinetics, Champaign, IL, 2002.
7. DeLorme, T. and A. Watkins, *Progressive Resistance Exercise,* Appleton-Century-Crofts, New York, 1951.
8. de Vries, H.A., *Physiology of Exercise for Physical Education and Athletics,* 4th ed., William C. Brown, Dubuque, IA, 1986.
9. Elliott, B.C. and C.A. Wood, Biomechanical principles, in *Textbook of Science and Medicine in Sport,* Bloomfield, J. P.A. Fricker, and K.D. Fitch, Eds., Human Kinetics, Champaign, IL, 1992.
10. Feigenbaum, M.S. and M.L. Pollack, Prescription of resistance training for health and disease, *Medicine and Science in Sports and Exercise,* 31, 38–45, 1999.
11. Fisher, A.G. and C.R. Jenson, *Scientific Basis of Athletic Conditioning,* 3rd ed., Lea and Febiger, Philadelphia, 1990.
12. Fleishman, E.A., *The Structure and Measurement of Physical Fitness,* Prentice-Hall, Englewood Cliffs, NJ, 1964.
13. Fox, E.L., R.W. Bowers, and M.L. Foss, *The Physiological Basis for Exercise and Sport,* 5th ed., Brown and Benchmark, Madison, WI, 1993.
14. Fox, S.I., *Human Physiology,* 3rd ed., William C. Brown, Dubuque, IA, 1990.

15. Graves, J.E. and M.L. Pollock, Understanding the physiological basis of muscular fitness, in *The Stairmaster's Fitness Handbook: A User's Guide to Exercise Testing and Prescription,* Peterson, J.A. and C.X. Bryant, Eds., Masters Press, Indianapolis, IN, 1992.
16. Hall, S.J., *Basic Biomechanics,* 2nd ed., Mosby Year Book, Inc., St. Louis, MO, 1995.
17. Hamill, J. and K.M. Knutzen, *Biomechanical Basis of Human Movement,* 2nd ed., Lippincott, Williams and Wilkins, Philadelphia, 2003.
18. Harman, E., The biomechanics of resistance exercise, in *Essentials of Strength Training and Conditioning,* 2nd ed., Baechle, T.R. and R.W. Earle, Eds., Human Kinetics, Champaign, IL, 2000.
19. Heyward, V.H., *Advanced Fitness Assessment and Exercise Prescription,* 2nd ed., Human Kinetics Books, Champaign, IL, 1991.
20. Howley, E.T. and B.D. Franks, *Health Fitness Instructors Handbook,* 4rth ed., Human Kinetics, Champaign, IL, 2003.
21. Hunter, G.R., Muscle physiology, in *Essentials of Strength Training and Conditioning,* 2nd ed., Baechle, T.R. and R.W. Earle, Eds., Human Kinetics, Champaign, IL, 2000.
22. Karp, J.R., Muscle fiber types and training, *Strength and Conditioning Journal,* National Strength and Conditioning Association, 23, 21–26, October, 2001.
23. Knudson, D.V., P. Magnusson, and M. McHugh. Current issues in flexibility fitness. *Research Digest,* President's Council on Physical Fitness and Sports, Series 3, No. 10, 1–8, June, 2000.
24. Kraemer, W.J., General adaptations to resistance and endurance training programs, in *Essentials of Strength Training and Conditioning,* 2nd ed., Baechle, T.R. and R.W. Earle, Eds., Human Kinetics, Champaign, IL, 2000.
25. Kraemer, W.J. and N.A. Ratamess, Progression and resistive training. *Research Digest,* The President's Council on Physical Fitness and Sports, Washington, DC, Series 6, No. 3, 1–8, September, 2005.
26. Lamb, D.R., *Physiology of Exercise; Responses and Adaptations,* 2nd ed., Macmillan, New York, 1984.
27. Lesmes, G.R. et al., Muscle strength and power changes during maximal isokinetic training, *Medicine and Science in Sports,* 10, 266–269, 1978.
28. Luber, R.L., *Skeletal Muscle Structure and Function: Implications for Rehabilitation and Sports Medicine,* Williams and Wilkins, Baltimore, 1992.
29. Luttgens, K., H. Deutsch, and N. Hamilton, *Kinesiology: Scientific Basis of Human Motion,* 8th ed., Brown and Benchmark, Madison, WI, 1992.
30. Marx, J.O. et al., Low volume circuit training versus high volume periodized resistance training in women, *Medicine and Science in Sports and Exercise,* 33, 635–643, 2001.
31. Maud, P.J. and C. Foster, *Physiological Assessment of Human Fitness,* Human Kinetics, Champaign, IL, 1995.
32. McArdle, W.D., F.I. Katch, and V.I. Katch, *Exercise Physiology: Energy, Nutrition, and Human Performance,* 6th ed., Lippincott, Williams, and Wilkins, Philadelphia, 2006.
33. Nelson, R.T. and W.D. Bandy, An update on flexibility, *Strength and Conditioning Journal,* National Strength and Conditioning Association, 27, 10–16, February, 2005.
34. Noakes, T., *Lore of Running,* 4rth ed., Human Kinetics, Champaign, IL, 2002.
35. Powers, S.K. and E.T. Howley, *Exercise Physiology: Theory and Application to Fitness and Performance,* 5th ed., McGraw-Hill, New York, 2004.
36. Robergs, R.A. and S.J. Keteyian, *Exercise Physiology: for Fitness, Performance, and Health,* 2nd ed., McGraw-Hill, New York, 2003.

37. Russell, B., D. Motlagh, and W.W. Ashley, Form follows function: how muscle shape is regulated by work, *Journal of Applied Physiology,* 88, 1127–1132, 2000.
38. Sale, D. and D. MacDougall, Specificity in strength training: a review of the coach and athlete, *Canadian Journal of Applied Sport Sciences,* 6, 87–92, 1981.
39. Vander, A.J., J.H. Sherman, and D.S. Luciano, *Human Physiology: The Mechanisms of Body Function,* 5th ed., McGraw-Hill, New York, 1990.
40. Williams, J.H., Normal musculoskeletal and neuromuscular anatomy, physiology, and responses to training, in *Clinical Exercise Physiology,* Hasson, S.M., Ed., Mosby Year Book, St. Louis, MO, 1994.
41. Wilmore, J.H. and D.L. Costill, *Physiology of Sport and Exercise,* 3rd ed., Human Kinetics, Champaign, IL, 2004.
42. Wilson, G.J., Strength and power in sports, in *Applied Anatomy and Biomechanics in Sport,* Bloomfield, J., T.R. Ackland, and B.C. Elliott, Eds., Blackwell Scientific Publications, Melbourne, Australia, 1994.
43. Wolkodoff, N., Training for strength, in *Fitness: Theory and Practice,* 2nd ed., Jordan, P., Ed., Aerobics and Fitness Association of America, Sherman Oaks, CA, 1995.

5 Aerobic and Anaerobic Conditioning

INTRODUCTION

The development of aerobic and anaerobic conditioning through physical training is significant to overall cardiovascular fitness and function. Metabolically, aerobic endurance provided by the oxidative system for long-distance performance is gained through work in the presence of oxygen, while anaerobic conditioning, made available through the use of the phosphagen or adenosine triphosphate–creatine phosphate (ATP-CP) and fast glycolytic or lactic acid systems for immediate and intensive physical activity, is attained through work without the presence of oxygen. The energy responses produced by these systems contribute to the resulting physiological work capacity of the body in regard to physical performance.

PHOSPHAGEN OR ADENOSINE TRIPHOSPHATE–CREATINE PHOSPHATE SYSTEM

The phosphagen system supplies the immediate anaerobic energy for physical work through the chemical breakdown of adenosine triphosphate (ATP) and creatine phosphate (CP) by the enzymatic actions of myosin ATPase and creatine kinase.[12,28] Myosin ATPase regulates the breakdown of ATP to adenosine diphosphate and phosphate (ADP+P) (Figure 5.1). Creatine kinase promotes the resynthesis of ATP from ADP and P and CP. The energy produced anaerobically only lasts for several seconds, making it necessary for ATP to be reformed in order for work to continue for longer periods of time. Physical work lasting longer than several seconds would depend upon further anaerobic (fast glycolysis) and/or aerobic (slow glycolysis) source processes.[23]

FAST GLYCOLYTIC OR LACTIC ACID SYSTEM

Intensive anaerobic energy is fueled primarily by glycogen and glucose through fast glycolytic processes (Figure 5.2).[9,26,31,55] Muscle glycogen breakdown occurs first, and then as levels become depleted, blood glucose becomes the preferred energy substrate. As glucose needs increase, liver glycogen is converted to glucose through glycogenolytic processes. Glucose in turn is degraded to pyruvic acid, resulting in an increase in lactic acid and fatigue levels. Intensive physical work can last for a

Adenosine Triphosphate ⟶ Adenosine Diphosphate and Phosphate = Energy Release

Creatine Phosphate ⟶ Creatine and Phosphate = Resynthesis of Adenosine Diphosphate and Phosphate to Adenosine Triphosphate

Adenosine Triphosphate ⟶ Adenosine Diphosphate and Phosphate = Energy Release

FIGURE 5.1 Phosphagen or adenosine triphosphate-creatine phosphate system.

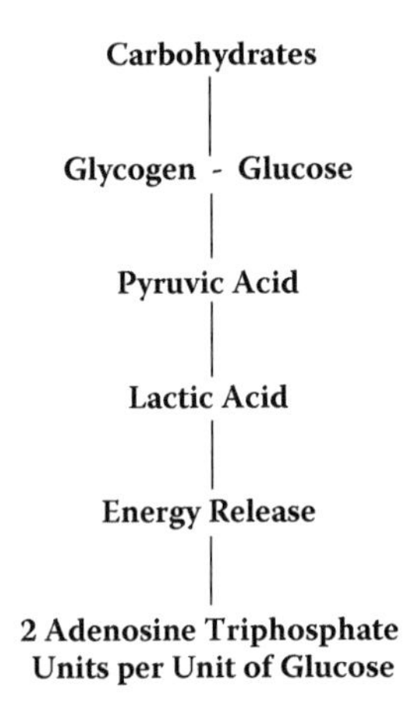

FIGURE 5.2 Fast glycolysis or lactic acid system.

short period of time.[17,18] This may be due to an increase in hydrogen ion and pH acidity levels, which in turn may inhibit muscle contraction processes.[12,28,37,53] At that point exhaustion occurs, since few ATP units have been produced. Excess amounts of lactic acid can generally be cleared from the blood if exercise intensity is lessened through Cori cycle processes and converted to pyruvic acid, which in turn can be reconverted to glucose in the liver. Light-to-moderate activity will promote clearance through oxidative phosphorylation processes.[11,48] Higher levels of lactic acid production have been related to work intensity and the greater use of fast muscle fiber types.[53] Fats and proteins play lesser roles during intensive physical work, but their use increases as exercise duration increases.

SLOW GLYCOLYTIC OR OXIDATIVE SYSTEM

Long-distance aerobic energy can be produced by the breakdown of carbohydrates, fats, and proteins to glucose and glycogen, glycerol and fatty acids, and amino acids, respectively (Figure 5.3). In the cellular organelles of the mitochondria, these nutrient substrates are sequentially converted to pyruvic acid and acetyl coenzyme A, if oxygen is available and the intensity of the exercise decreases, and go through Krebs cycle processes. Molecules of the reduced forms of nicotinamide adenine dinucle-

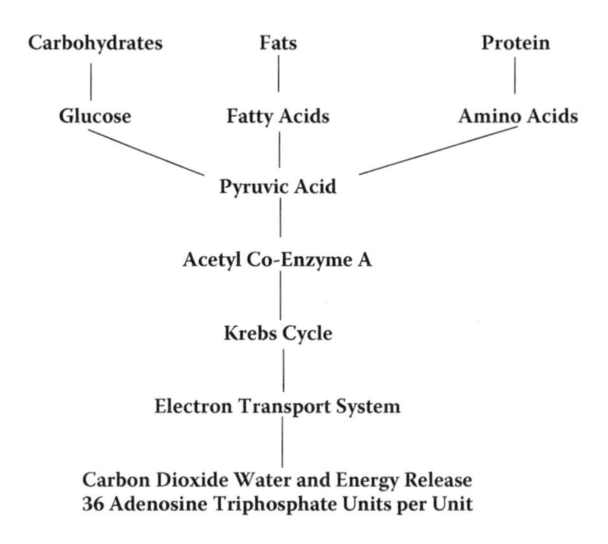

FIGURE 5.3 Slow glycolysis or oxidative system.

otide (NADH) and flavin adenine dinucleotide (FADH), electron and hydrogen carriers formed in the Krebs cycle, pass on the hydrogen to the electron transport chain. In the electron transport chain, the hydrogen ions are processed through cytochrome degradation fueled by NAD, FAD, and coenzyme Q, another electron carrier, synthesizing ADP and P to ATP and water.[28] Thirty-six ATP units are produced in the process, allowing for long periods of moderate physical work. Fats and carbohydrates are predominantly used in the process. During aerobic exercise the lactic acid that is produced can readily be cleared from the blood. All three energy systems work in interactive conjunction with one another, utilizing appropriate oxidative and glycolytic metabolic processes in greater and/or lesser degrees dependent upon bodily needs in response to exercise. (Figure 5.4)

MUSCLE FIBER TYPES

There are basically two muscle fiber types, slow twitch and fast twitch (Table 5.1). Slow-twitch fibers are slow in contraction speed, high in fatigue resistance, and high in aerobic capacity. Fast-twitch fibers are fast in contraction speed, low in fatigue resistance, and high in anaerobic capacity. Twitch refers to contraction response to stimuli. Slow-twitch fibers are oxidative in nature and are used for endurance activities, whereas fast-twitch fibers are glycolytic in nature and are used for short and intense activities.

Muscle fiber types are genetically determined and are classified according to their morphological, metabolic, mechanical, and histochemical properties.[26,35] Type I (slow oxidative) fibers are smaller in size, produce less force, possess more mitochondria and enzymes to convert fats and carbohydrates to carbon dioxide and water, and transport more oxygen than do fast-twitch fibers.[37] Two subdivisions of fast-twitch fibers have been identified.[15,56] Type II A and Type II B fibers have been found to range from fast oxidative/glycolytic to fast glycolytic, providing limited aerobic to

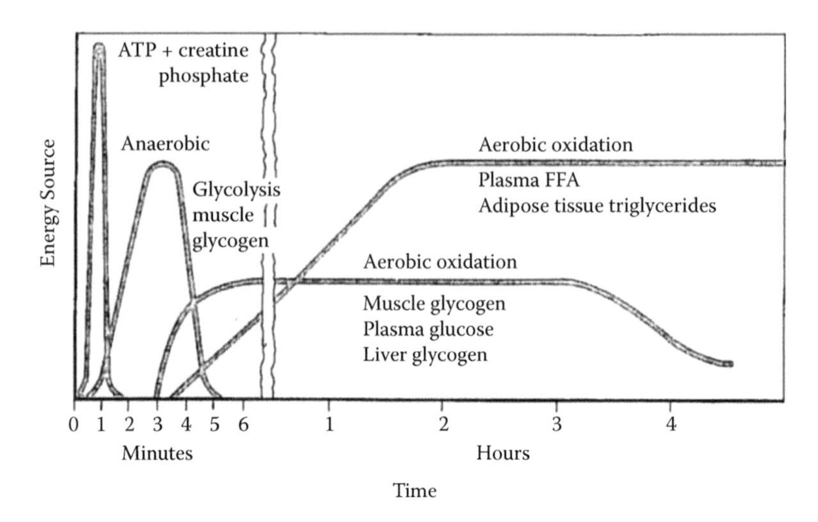

FIGURE 5.4 Utilization of energy sources. (From Berne, R. M. and M. N. Levy, *Physiology,* 3rd ed., Mosby Yearbook, St. Louis, 1993. With permission from Elsevier.)

TABLE 5.1
Skeletal Muscle Fiber Types

Fiber Types	Fiber Contraction Speed	Oxidative Glycolytic	Fatigue Onset
I	Slow	Oxidative	Slow
IIa	Intermediate	Oxidative	Fast
		Glycolytic	Intermediate
IIIb	Fast	Glycolytic	Fast

[a] Oxidative – oxygen utilization for endurance exercises.
[b] Glycolytic – nonoxygen utilization for short intense exercises.

totally anaerobic distributions of energy utilization. In reference to muscle fiber type distribution, endurance athletes tend to have greater percentages of slow-twitch fibers, whereas nonendurance athletes tend to have more fast-twitch fibers, on the average.

Muscle fiber types also have the potential for optimal development within designated genetic limits.[56] Endurance training results in the increase of mitochondrial concentration and oxidative enzyme levels, while nonendurance training produces an increase in muscle size and glycolytic enzyme levels.[27] In reference to the ability of muscle fibers to change their endowed characteristics, early studies basically showed that such conversion was not possible.[21] However, some studies have reported slow- and fast-twitch muscle fiber interchanges following increased physical training. Current research indicates such conversions can occur but are genetically limited.[27,28,44,48,57] Phenotypically however, such interchanges may occur due to the myosin isoform ratio distributive pattern in muscle fibers.[10,54] Fast- and slow-twitch muscle fibers contain different amounts of myosin isoforms. These isoform

Frequency	Most Days of the Week
Intensity	50 – 75% 70 – 85%
Duration	30 – 60 Minutes

FIGURE 5.5 Exercise prescription. (Adapted from Your Guide to Physical Activity and Your Heart, National Institutes of Health, National Heart, Lung, and Blood Institute, NIH Publication No. 06-5714, June, 2006.)

levels have been reported to be dependent on the training program utilized.[10,54] The fast-twitch myosin isoforms would be increased during intensity training, and the slow-twitch myosin isoforms would be increased during endurance exercise.

PRINCIPLES OF TRAINING

The basic cardiovascular training principles are frequency (number), intensity (degree), duration (length), and specificity (type) (Figure 5.5).[42] According to the American College of Sports Medicine,[2] three to five workouts per week, 50/60 to 90% of maximum heart rate, and 20 to 60 min or a minimum of 20 to 30 min of continuous exercise time are advocated for the development and maintenance of cardiovascular health. Exercise activities relative to mode, including walking, jogging, running, bicycling, swimming, and dancing, which utilize the large muscles of body, are continuous in nature and are aerobically oriented.

In reference to frequency, three to five workouts per week have been found to significantly increase aerobic capacity.[8,10] Less than two workouts per week seems to limit cardiovascular development and maintenance.[47,52] This was shown in a study done by Gettman et al.,[24] in which they found significant differences between one-, three-, and five-day training programs over a period of 20 weeks. The results showed 8, 13, and 17% increases in aerobic capacities for the groups, respectively.

The intensity of exercise refers to work level. The determination of work level can be based on maximum oxygen consumption. Since maximum oxygen consumption is difficult to assess without laboratory testing, heart rate can be used.[2,25] Heart rate can generally be determined through the use of the formula 220 minus your age times the submaximal training rate desired.[8,29] Target heart rate zones according to age levels for the determination of appropriate work range levels have been developed (Figure 5.6).[42] These ranges extend from 60 to 90% of submaximal heart rate levels. Work below the 60% range, which is designated as the minimal threshold level, would not significantly improve cardiovascular endurance, while work within and above the target range zones would significantly increase aerobic capacity levels.[2] Karvonen et al.[30] found significant differences in the training of young men at intensity levels below the heart rate of 135 and above the heart rate of 153 beats per minute relative to aerobic improvement. Recently, however, lower exercise

Age	Target Heart Rate Zone 50/70 – 85%	Maximum Heart Rates
20	100/140 – 170	200
25	98/137 – 166	195
30	95/133 – 162	190
35	93/130 – 157	185
40	90/136 – 153	180
45	88/123 – 149	175
50	85/119 – 145	170
55	83/116 – 139	165
60	80/112 – 136	160
65	78/108 – 132	155
70	75/105 - 128	150

Formula Utilization - 220 – Age = Maximum Heart Rate

FIGURE 5.6 Maximal and submaximal heart rates and target zones for different age levels. (Adapted from Your Guide to Physical Activity and Your Heart. National Institutes of Health, National Heart, Lung, and Blood Institute, NIH Publication No. 06-5714, June, 2006.)

intensity work ranges of 50 to 60% have also been designated.[29,47,52] Based on recent research on the values of moderate exercise, both the American College of Sports Medicine[2] and the American Heart Association[18] have published position papers in this regard. Continuous forms of exercise, such as walking, hiking, jogging, cycling, swimming, and participation in other similar sports activities performed within lower moderate (40 to 60%) target ranges, have proven to be beneficial relative to aerobic capacity, health, disease prevention, and longevity.[8,22] In this regard, Duncan et al. found high (65–75%) and moderate (45–55%) intensity aerobic exercise combined with high-frequency workouts resulted in cardiorespiratory improvement over a period of 24 months.[14] The study included 30 minutes of walking five to seven days per week.

Perceived exertion rate during exercise has also been used as an indicator of exercise intensity (Table 5.2).[45] Number scales developed by Borg[5] of 6 to 20 and 1 to 10 interval levels descriptive of increasing effort ranges have been available for use in this regard (Table 5.3). These scales have been reported to be significantly related to heart rate and aerobic conditioning.[2] The Borg Scales can be used as representative indicators of graded quantitative exercise intensity and as guides to the changes that occur with the conditioning effects of physical work endurance. As guides, the scales can also be used at preferred training exertion submaximal and maximal aerobic capacity levels by athletes (Table 5.4).[41]

The duration of exercise refers to the length of activity time. Twenty to sixty minutes of continuous exercise is advocated within intensity range levels.[2] Milesis et al.,[39] in a training study of men exercising for 15, 30, and 45 min per workout session, found aerobic improvement to be 8.5, 16.1, and 16.8%, respectively, for the three groups. Exercise training at lower intensity levels but longer duration will result in similar aerobic capacity increases when compared to shorter and more intensive workout ranges.[8]

TABLE 5.2
Classification of Intensity of Exercise Based on 30 to 60 Minutes of Endurance Training

Relative Intensity			
HRmax	VO_2max or HRmax Reserve	Rating of Perceived Exertion	Classification of Intensity
<35%	<30%	<10	Very light
35–59%	30–49%	10–11	Light
60–79%	50–74	12–13	Moderate
80–89%	75–84%	14–16	Heavy
≥90%	≥85%	>16	Very heavy

Source: Adapted from Pollock, M.L. and J.H. Wilmore, *Exercise in Health and Disease: Evaluation and Prescription for Prevention and Rehabilitation,* 2nd ed., W. B. Saunders, Philadelphia, 1990. With permission from Elsevier.

TABLE 5.3
Least Effort

Rating	Zone
6	
7 very, very light	
8	
9 very light	
10	
11 fairly light	
12	Endurance Training Zone
13 somewhat hard	
14	
15 hard	
16	Strength Training Zone
17 very hard	
18	
19 very, very hard	
20	
Maximum Effort	

Source: The Borg Category Rating Scale adapted from Exercise: A Guide from the National Institute on Aging. National Institutes of Health. National Institute on Aging. NIH Publication No. 01-4258, April, 2004. With permission.

TABLE 5.4
Aerobic Capacity of Elite Athletes

	Men (ml/kg/min)	Women (ml/kg/min)
Endurance sports		
Long distance running	75–80	65–70
Cross-country skiing	75–78	65–70
Biathlon	75–78	—
Road cycling	70–75	60–65
Middle-distance running	70–75	65–68
Skating	65–72	55–60
Orienteering	65–72	60–65
Swimming	60–70	55–60
Rowing	65–69	60–64
Track racing	65–70	55–60
Canoeing	60–68	50–55
Walking	60–65	55–60
Games		
Football (soccer)	50–57	—
Handball	55–60	48–52
Ice hockey	55–60	—
Volleyball	55–60	48–52
Basketball	50–55	40–45
Tennis	48–52	40–45
Table tennis	40–45	38–42
Combative sports		
Boxing	60–65	—
Wrestling	60–65	—
Judo	55–60	50–55
Fencing	45–50	40–45
Power sports		
Sprint (200 m track)	55–60	45–50
Sprint track and field (100 m, 200 m)	48–52	43–47
Long jump	50–55	45–50
Competition consisting of several events (decathlon, septathlon)	60–65	50–55
Nordic combination (15 km ski walking and ski jumping)	60–65	—
Weight lifting	40–50	—
Discus throwing, shot putting	40–45	35–40
Javelin throwing	45–50	42–47
Pole vaulting	45–50	—
Ski jumping	40–45	—
Technical-acrobatic sports		
Down-hill skiing (Alpine disciplines)	60–65	48–53
Figure skating	50–55	45–50

TABLE 5.4 *(Continued)*
Aerobic Capacity of Elite Athletes

	Men (ml/kg/min)	Women (ml/kg/min)
Gymnastics	45–50	40–45
Rhythmic gymnastics	—	40–45
Sailing	50–55	45–50
Shooting	40–45	35–40

Source: From Neumann, G., in *The Olympic Book of Sports Medicine,* Vol. 1, Dirix, A., H. G. Knuttgen, and K. Tittle, Eds., Blackwell Scientific Publications, Oxford, 1988. With permission.

The total amount of work done would determine overall fitness improvement levels. Activities of longer duration would be conducted at lower intensity ranges, while those of shorter duration would be performed at higher intensity ranges when energy costs were held constant. Within this frame of reference, De Busk et al. found three 10-min moderate intensity workouts also effectively demonstrated aerobic development.[13] Warm-up and cool-down periods preceding and following exercise time should be included for the possible prevention of injury.

Specificity refers to the metabolic and muscular changes that occur due to the mode of training adopted. Generally, studies have demonstrated that the metabolic changes resulting from training are aerobically and anaerobically specific to the type of exercise undergone.[38,52] Aerobic training is related to long-term oxidative energy system development, while anaerobic training is related to short-term glycolytic adaptations in the body.[20,48] Even though there is interaction between the two energy systems, little transfer occurs relative to type of training. Bouchard et al.,[4] in their study on aerobic capacity in relation to leg cycling, arm cranking, uphill treadmill, walking, and bench stepping training methods among untrained men, found that treadmill walking elicited the highest maximal oxidative responses.

In reference to muscular specificity and training method, similar results have been observed. Studies have generally demonstrated that there is little transfer between muscle groups from one part of the body to another.[48] This may be due to the type of muscle fibers used (slow twitch or fast twitch) and the recruitment pattern of muscle groups. In a study by Fox et al.,[19] male college students were trained on bicycle ergometers in reference to submaximal interval arm and leg pedaling for 5 weeks. The results were specific in nature and were related to the trained arm or leg utilized.

TRAINING PROGRAMS

The basic training programs are those of continuous, interval, and fartlek or speed play.[49] Continuous programs refer to endurance types of training relative to the raising and maintenance of heart rate within designated target ranges. Interval programs are intermittent in nature relative to vigorous and moderate combinations of activity that are preplanned over set distances. In this regard, heart rate would be raised and lowered as determined by activity levels. Fartlek or speed play programs are similar to interval, but differ in reference to set distances of varying intensities.

All three programs can incorporate combined workouts that are aerobic and anaerobic in nature and include training that is short, moderate, or long relative to activity length, and slow, moderate, or fast in reference to intensity of effort. Aerobic programs are usually endurance oriented relative to distance in order to increase oxidative capacity.[56] Interval and fartlek programs are usually intensity oriented and are designed to increase anaerobic capacity. Pace, hill, and speed training methods have been utilized for such energy systems development. Repeated short distances and speed are specifically designed to condition the immediate ATP-PC system, while repeated intermediate distances and speed are designated for lactic acid system development. Both of these systems are anaerobic in nature. Long distances and slow speed are specifically geared to condition the oxygen-supplied aerobic system of energy.

EFFECTS OF CARDIOVASCULAR TRAINING PROGRAMS

Cardiovascular endurance training programs bring about a variety of chronic changes in the body that result in greater energy production and improved physical performance (Table 5.5). These changes include cardiac, circulatory, respiratory, muscular, and body-composition responses that are made to training of this nature.

The metabolic changes that result from training include the aerobic and anaerobic effects of conditioning. Aerobically, oxidative capacity is increased due to increases in mitochondrial size and number, in Krebs cycle and electron transport system enzymatic reactions, and in carbohydrate and fat oxidation.[1,3,21,27,40,44,48,52,57] Anaerobically, muscular stores of adenosine triphosphate and phosphocreatine are increased, and glycolytic enzymatic reactions occur faster, resulting in greater nonoxidative endurance.[21,37,48,57] An anaerobic endurance increase is also related to a decreased lactic acid accumulation, which would in essence delay the onset of fatigue.[32,37,48]

The cardiovascular changes that result from training are mainly centered in cardiac and circulatory adaptations to exercise. Cardiac size and volume, and cardiac stroke volume and output are increased, while cardiac working and resting rates are decreased.[1,7,21,36,50] Cardiac hypertrophy is characterized by a larger ventricle cavity, which would house a greater volume of blood and in turn increase the stroke volume and output from the heart during training and at rest.[19,21,37] In essence, the heart becomes larger, more efficient, and more effective because of the necessary training adaptations made in response to vigorous exercise. There are also increases in hemoglobin, myoglobin, and blood volume.[21,27,36,37,50,51] These increases result in a greater amount of oxygen diffused to the mitochondria and prove to be significant to aerobic capacity enhancement.[43,44,57] Blood lipids and blood pressure are also affected by endurance training. High-density-lipoprotein cholesterol is increased, while low-density-lipoprotein cholesterol is decreased.[29,33,34] Triglyceride levels are

TABLE 5.5
The Effects of Aerobic Endurance on Health and Fitness Variables

Variable	Resistance exercise
Bone Mineral Density	↑↑
Body Composition	
%fat	↓
LBM	↑↑
Strength	↑↑↑
Glucose Metabolism	
Insulin response to glucose challenge	↓↓
Basal insulin levels	↓
Insulin Sensitivity	↑↑
Serum lipids	
HDL	↑↔
LDL	↓↔
Resting heart rate	↔
Stroke volume	↔
Blood Pressure at rest	
Systolic	↔
Diastolic	↓↔
VO_2 max	↑
Endurance Time	↑↑
Physical function	↑↑↑
Basal metabolism	↑↑

Source: Adapted from Pollock, M. L. and K. R. Vincent, Resistance Training for Health. The President's Council on Physical Fitness and Sports Research Digest, Series 2, No. 8, December, 1996.

also decreased.[19,33] Studies have also shown that moderate to moderate-intensive endurance exercise would decrease blood pressure levels.[6,16,49]

Respiratory responses to exercise result in increased tidal volume, breathing frequency, minute ventilation and efficiency, larger lung volume, and greater oxygen–carbon dioxide diffusion capacity.[21,50,55] The increases in both tidal volume and breathing frequency result in greater maximal minute ventilation capacity and an increase in ventilatory efficiency.[21,52] Lung volume is also enhanced due to training and increased pulmonary function.[21,52] The increase in lung volume, in turn, results in greater diffusion capacity both at rest and during exercise.[21]

The muscular changes that occur as a result of endurance training generally include increases in skeletal muscle hypertrophy, capillary density, and muscle fiber type capacity.[43,56,57] Skeletal muscle hypertrophy increases due to training are related to enhanced capillary density.[7] These increases result in muscle fiber development and greater blood flow, which in turn increase the amount of oxygen, glycogen, and fatty acids brought to the working muscles.[19] In regard to muscle fiber type changes, endurance training enhances both the oxidative and glycolytic capacities in slow-twitch and fast-twitch fibers, respectively.[21]

The body composition changes generally include the lean and fat tissue adaptations that occur as a result of endurance training. In response to such exercise, there is little or no increase in lean body tissue and a decrease in body fat.[1,32] Total body weight may also be decreased. Weight loss would be dependent on exercise intensity and duration, as well as caloric intake and expenditure.[19,48]

PRE-ENTRANCE PROGRAM CONSIDERATIONS

Training considerations taken prior to program implementation include those of age, sex, health status, previous and present levels of conditioning, motivation, and goals.[2,17,29,42]

1. Age and gender — Exercise programs should be based on individualized needs relative to health and fitness considerations.
2. Health status — Medical examinations form the basis for the factor of health status, which would in turn determine the amount, type, and rate of exercise prescription.
3. Previous conditioning experiences and present levels of condition — Based on past training experiences, present conditioning levels will reflect the frequency, intensity, and duration of the exercise program to be implemented.
4. Motivation — Each person is motivated differently relative to exercise needs, perception levels, learning abilities, and self-discipline regarding training. Such factors may result in strong or diminished drives toward program adoption.
5. Goals and measurement — Sequence, rate of progression, frequency, intensity, and duration of exercise goals should be predetermined to some degree and periodic assessments made.

SUMMARY

In summary, research studies in the area of aerobic and anaerobic endurance have demonstrated the following results:

1. The development of aerobic and anaerobic endurance through physical training is significant to overall cardiovascular fitness and function.
2. Aerobic and anaerobic energy systems work in interactive conjunction with one another, utilizing appropriate oxidative and glycolytic metabolic processes in greater and/or lesser degrees, depending on bodily needs in response to exercise.
3. The phosphagen system provides an immediate anaerobic form of energy for several seconds through the breakdown of adenosine triphosphate and creatine phosphate.

4. The fast glycolytic system provides an intensive anaerobic form of energy for a short period of time through the breakdown of glucose to pyruvic acid and lactic acid.
5. The oxidative system provides an aerobic duration form of energy for an unlimited time period through the degradation of pyruvic acid to acetyl Coenzyme A.
6. Slow- and fast-twitch muscle fiber types are genetically determined. Slow-twitch fibers are slow in contraction speed, high in fatigue resistance, and high in aerobic capacity. Fast-twitch fibers are fast in contraction speed, low in fatigue resistance, and high in anaerobic capacity.
7. The basic principles of training are those of frequency (number), intensity (degree), duration (length), and specificity (type).
8. Perceived exertion rating systems can be used as indicators of exercise intensity.
9. The basic training programs are those of distance, interval, and fartlek or speed play.
10. Cardiovascular endurance training programs bring about a variety of chronic changes in the body that result in greater energy production and improved physical performance. These changes include cardiac, circulatory, respiratory, muscular, and body composition responses that are made to training of this nature.
11. Training considerations taken prior to program implementation include those of age, sex, health status, previous and present levels of conditioning, motivation, and goals.

GLOSSARY

Actin Thin protein filament found in myofibrils that interacts with myosin in muscle contraction processes

Acetyl coenzyme A A substrate produced by the breakdown of fat to fatty acids

Adenosine diphosphate Chemical compound that interacts with inorganic phosphate to form adenosine triphosphate

Adenosine triphosphatase Protein enzyme catalyst involved in muscle contraction processes

Adenosine triphosphate/creatine phosphate Immediate energy compound sources involved in muscle contraction processes

Aerobic conditioning Physical work done in the presence of oxygen

Amino acids The basic components of proteins that contain amino and acid groups attached to central carbon atoms with different side chains

Anaerobic conditioning Physical work done without the presence of oxygen

Coenzyme Q Electron carrier active in transport chain processes

Cori cycle The lactic acid conversion to pyruvic acid, which in turn is reconverted to glucose in the liver

Creatine kinase Promotes the resynthesis of ATP from ADP and P and CP

Distance training Refers to continuous types of training relative to the raising and maintenance of heart rate within designated target ranges
Duration Refers to the work length of the exercise session
Electron transport system The chemical process through which adenosine triphosphate is resynthesized in the mitochondria
Energy metabolism The biochemical processes involved in the production of energy
Fartlek training Speed play training without set distances of varying activity
Fast-twitch muscle fiber types Muscle fibers that are anaerobic, fast contracting, and fast fatiguing
Fats Compounds that contain carbon, hydrogen, and oxygen and are classified as triglycerides, phospholipids, and cholesterol
Flavin adenine dinucleotide Electron and hydrogen carrier
Frequency Refers to the number of exercise sessions per week
Glucose The basic carbohydrate unit that serves as a major energy fuel
Glycogen The stored form of glucose in muscle and liver tissue
Glycogenolysis The conversion of glycogen to glucose
Glycolysis (fast) Anaerobic process involved in the breakdown of glucose to lactic acid
Hemoglobin Chemical component that binds to oxygen and contains iron and protein
High-density lipoproteins Lipoproteins that are small in size, dense in weight, and are the main carriers of cholesterol from body tissues
Intensity Refers to the work level of the exercise session
Interval training Intermittent training relative to vigorous and moderate combinations of activity that are preplanned over set distances
Krebs cycle The process through which carbohydrates, fats, and protein are converted to water and carbon dioxide in the formation of energy
Lactic acid Anaerobic end product of glucose conversion to lactate
Low-density lipoproteins Lipoproteins that contain mostly cholesterol and are the prime carriers of this sterol to body tissues
Minute ventilation The amount of air inhaled or exhaled in each minute
Mitochondria Energy-producing cellular organelles
Motor neuron Pertains to nerve cells involved in the innervation of muscle tissue
Muscle hypertrophy Increase in muscle size and diameter as a result of resistance training
Myoglobin Protein that binds to oxygen
Myosin Thick protein filament found in myofibrils that interacts with actin in muscle contraction processes
Myosin adenosine triphosphatase Regulates the breakdown of ATP to ADP and P
Myosin distributive isoform ratio percentages Possible ratio conversions in fast- and slow-twitch muscle fibers
Nicotinamide adenine dinucleotide Electron and hydrogen carrier
Oxidative system (slow glycolysis) Aerobic process involved in the interaction of inorganic phosphate and adenosine diphosphate to form adenosine triphosphate

pH levels Acidity levels during intensive anaerobic exercise
Polarization/depolarization Electrical activity processes generated in nerve and muscle tissue during reversal of positive and negative sodium and potassium ions
Pyruvic acid A carbon molecule that is a resultant of glucose breakdown
Slow-twitch muscle fiber types Muscle fibers that are aerobic, slow contracting, and fast fatiguing
Specificity Aerobic/anaerobic conditioning through utilization of designated training programs
Tidal volume Amount of air inhaled and exhaled in each breath taken
Triglycerides Fat compounds that contain glycerol and three fatty acids

REFERENCES

1. Abernathy, B. et al., *The Biophysical Foundations of Human Movement,* 2nd ed., Human Kinetics, Baltimore, 2005.
2. American College of Sports Medicine, *ACSM's Guidelines for Exercise Testing and Prescription,* 7th ed., Lippincott, Williams, and Wilkins, Philadelphia, 2005.
3. Astrand, P.O., K. Rodahl, and H.A. Dahl. *Textbook of Work Physiology,* 4th ed., Human Kinetics, Champaign, IL, 2003.
4. Bouchard, C. et al., Specificity of maximal aerobic power, *European Journal of Applied Physiology,* 40, 85–93, 1979.
5. Borg, G.A.V., Psychological bases of physical exertion, *Medicine and Science in Sports and Exercise,* 14, 377–381, 1982.
6. Boyer, J., and F. Kasch, Exercise therapy in hypertensive men, *Journal of the American Medical Association,* 211, 1668–1671, 1970.
7. Bowers, R.W. and E.L. Fox, *Sports Physiology,* 3rd ed., William C. Brown, Dubuque, IA, 1992.
8. Braun, L.T. Exercise physiology and cardiovascular fitness, *Nursing Clinics of North America,* 26, 135–147, 1991.
9. Brouns, F. and C. Cargill, *Essentials of Sports Nutrition,* 2nd ed., John Wiley and Sons, New York, 2002.
10. Brown, S.P., W.C. Miller, and J.M. Eason, *Exercise Physiology: Basis of Human Movement in Health and Disease,* Lippincott, Williams, and Wilkins, Baltimore, 2006.
11. Cerny, F.J. and H.W. Burton, *Exercise Physiology for Health Care Professionals,* Human Kinetics, Champaign, IL, 2001.
12. Craig, B.W., Does muscle pH affect performance? *Strength and Conditioning Journal,* National Strength and Conditioning Association, 26, 24–25, December, 2004.
13. De Busk, R.F. et al., Training effects of long versus short bouts of exercise in healthy subjects, *American Journal of Cardiology,* 65, 1010–1013, 1990.
14. Duncan, G.F. et al., Prescribing exercise at varied levels of intensity and frequency: a randomized trial, *Archives of Internal Medicine,* 165, 2362–2369, November 14, 2005.
15. Enoka, R.M., *Neuromechanics of Human Movement,* 3rd ed., Human Kinetics, Champaign, IL, 2001.
16. Fagard, R.H., Exercise characteristics and the blood pressure response to dynamic physical training, *Medicine and Science in Sports and Exercise,* 33, S484–492; 2001.

17. Fletcher, G.F. and J.F. Trejo, Why and how to prescribe exercise: overcoming the barriers, *Cleveland Clinic Journal of Medicine,* 72, 645–656, August, 2005.
18. Fletcher, G.F. et al., American Heart Association Scientific Council: position statement on exercise, *Circulation,* 86, 340–344, July, 1992.
19. Fox, E., D. McKenzie, and K. Cohen, Specificity of training: metabolic and circulatory responses, *Medicine and Science in Sports,* 7, 83, 1975.
20. Fox, E.L. *Sport Physiology,* 2nd ed., Saunders College Publishing, New York, 1984.
21. Fox, E.L., R.W. Bowers, and M.L. Foss, *The Physiological Basis for Exercise and Sport,* 5th ed., Brown and Benchmark, Madison, WI, 1993.
22. Franks, B.D., Personalizing physical activity prescription, The President's Council on Physical Fitness and Sports Research Digest, Series 2, No. 9, 1–8, March, 1997.
23. Gastin, P.B., Energy system interaction and relative contribution during maximal exercise, *Sports Medicine,* 31, 725–741, 2001.
24. Gettmen, L.R., M.L. Pollock, J.L. Durstine, A. Ward, J. Ayres, and A.C. Linnerud, Physiological responses of men to 1, 3, and 5 day per week training programs, *Research Quarterly,* 47, 638–646, 1976.
25. Gibson, S.B., S.G. Gerberich, and A.S. Leon, Writing the exercise prescription: an individualized approach, *The Physician and Sports Medicine,* 11, 87–100, 1983.
26. Hamill, J. and K.M. Knutzen, *Biomechanical Basis of Human Movement,* 2nd ed., Lippincott, Williams, and Wilkins, Philadelphia, 2003.
27. Housh, T.J., D.J. Housh, and H.A. de Vries, *Applied Exercise and Sport Physiology,* Holcomb Hathaway Publishers, Scottsdale, AZ, 2003.
28. Houston, M.E., *Biochemistry Primer for Exercise Science,* 2nd ed., Human Kinetics, Champaign, IL, 2001.
29. Howley, E.T. and B.D. Franks, *Health Fitness Instructor's Handbook,* 4rth ed., Human Kinetics, Champaign, IL, 2003.
30. Karvonen, M., E. Kentala, and O. Musta, The effects of training heart rate: a longitudinal study, *Annales Medicinae Experimentalis Biologiae Fenniae,* 35, 307–315, 1957.
31. Knuttgen, H.G. What is exercise? *Physician and Sportsmedicine,* 31, 31–39, March, 2003.
32. Kraemer, W.J. General adaptations to resistance and endurance training programs, in *Essentials of Strength Training and Conditioning,* 2nd ed., Baechle, T.R. and R.W. Earle, Eds., Human Kinetics, Champaign, IL, 2000.
33. Kwiterovich, P.O., *The Johns Hopkins Complete Guide for Preventing and Reversing Heart Disease,* Prima Publishing, Rocklen, California, 1993.
34. Leon, A.S. and O.A. Sanchez, Response of blood lipids to exercise training alone or combined with dietary intervention, *Medicine and Science in Sports and Exercise,* 33, s502–515, 2001.
35. Levangie, P.K. and C.C. Norkin, *Joint Structure and Function: A Comprehensive Analysis,* 4th ed., F.A. Davis Company, Philadelphia, 2005.
36. McArdle, W.D., F.I. Katch, and V.L. Katch, *Essentials of Exercise Physiology,* 3rd ed., Lippincott, Williams, and Wilkins, Philadelphia, 2005.
37. McArdle, W.D., F.I. Katch, and V.L. Katch, *Exercise Physiology: Energy, Nutrition, and Human Performance,* 6th ed., Lippincott, Williams, and Wilkins, Philadelphia, 2006.
38. McCafferty, W.B. and S.M. Howath, Specificity of exercise and specificity training, *Research Quarterly,* 48, 358–371, 1977.

39. Milesis, C.A. et al., Effects of different durations of training on cardiorespiratory function, body composition, and serum lipids, *Research Quarterly,* 47, 716–725, 1976.
40. Morgan, T., L. et al., Effects of long-term exercise on human muscle mitochondria, in *Muscle Metabolism During Exercise,* Pernow, B. and B. Saltin, Plenum Press, New York, 1971.
41. Morgan, W.P., Psychological components of effort sense, *Medicine and Science in Sports and Exercise,* 26, 1071–1077, 1994.
42. National Institutes of Health, National Heart, Lung, and Blood Institute, *Exercise and Your Heart: A Guide to Physical Activity,* 1989.
43. Noakes, T. *Lore of Running,* 4th ed., Human Kinetics, Champaign, IL, 2002.
44. Plowman, S.A., and D.L. Smith, *Exercise Physiology for Health, Fitness, and Performance,* 2nd ed., Benjamin Cummings, San Francisco, 2003.
45. Pollock, M.L. and J.H. Wilmore, *Exercise in Health and Disease: Evaluation and Prescription for Prevention and Rehabilitation,* 2nd ed., W.B. Saunders, Philadelphia, 1991.
46. Pollock, M.L., M.S. Fiegenbaume, and W.F. Brechue, Exercise prescription for physical fitness, *Quest,* 47, 320–337, 1995.
47. Pollock, M.L. et al., Effects of frequency and duration of training on attrition and incidence of injury, *Medicine and Science in Sports,* 9, 31–36, 1977.
48. Powers, S.K., and E.T. Howley, *Exercise Physiology: Theory and Application to Fitness and Performance,* 5th ed., McGraw-Hill, New York, 2004.
49. Rankinen, T. and C. Bouchard, Dose–response issues concerning the relations between regular physical activity and health, *Research Digest,* President's Council on Physical Fitness and Sports, Series 3, No. 18, 1–8, 2002.
50. Robergs, R.A. and S.J. Keteyian, *Fundamentals of Exercise Physiology for Fitness, Performance, and Health,* 2nd ed., McGraw-Hill, New York, 2003.
51. Sharkey, B.J. and S.E. Gaskill, *Sport Physiology for Coaches,* Human Kinetics, Champaign, IL, 2006.
52. Skinner, J.S., General principles of exercise prescription, in *Exercise Testing and Exercise Prescription for Special Cases: Theoretical Basis and Clinical Application,* 3rd ed., Skinner, J.S., Ed., Lippincott, Williams, and Wilkins, Philadelphia, 2005.
53. Stone, M.H. and M.S. Conley, Bioenergetics, in *Essentials of Strength Training and Conditioning,* Baechle, T.R., Ed., Human Kinetics, Champaign, IL, 1994.
54. Virer, A. and M. Virer, Nature of training effects, in *Exercise and Sport Science,* Garrett, W.E. and D.T. Kirkendall, Eds., Lippincott, Williams, and Wilkins, Philadelphia, 1999.
55. Wildman, R.E.C. and B.S. Miller, *Sports and Fitness Nutrition,* Wadsworth, Thomson Learning, Belmont, CA, 2004.
56. Wilmore, J.H. and D.L. Costill, *Physiology of Sport and Exercise,* 3rd ed., Human Kinetics, Champaign, IL, 2004.
57. Wilmore, J.H. Aerobic exercise and endurance: improving fitness for health benefits, *The Physician and Sports Medicine,* 31, No. 5, May, 2003.

Part Three

Motor Learning and Motor Control

6 Motor Learning and Motor Control

INTRODUCTION

Motor learning and motor control can be described generally as two interconnected fields of study concerned with the processes and mechanisms underlying the learning and acquirement of movement skills. Two parallel research areas of interest have historically been advanced during this time, namely the concepts of generality and specificity. Early studies were focused on general and specific motor abilities, while recent studies have been centered on open and closed looped motor programs and dynamic and exploratory search systems. In addition, motor learning and motor control are the interconnected areas of study that provide the processes and mechanisms underlying the learning and acquiring of motor skills.

GENERALITY AND SPECIFICITY

The generality and specificity of motor ability in theory and in practice has been studied by many researchers in the fields of physical education and athletics. In earlier studies, motor ability was regarded as being general in nature and in scope (Table 6.1). Component abilities were established in the areas of muscular strength, muscular endurance, flexibility, power, speed, agility, coordination, and stamina, and were representative of inherited and acquired skills which were considered to be transferable in relation to physical performance.[8,10,48,62,66] Tests and measures were developed and applied as performance determinants to predictive proficiency in athletic activities. Later studies in this field of research, however, disputed such general findings in regard to motor ability. Subsequent investigations were more demonstrative of the specificities in movement parameters (Table 6.2).[4,5,9,29,69] These later theories were more neuromotor centered and were considered to be independent and nontransferable relative to the performance specificities derived from undertaken physical tasks.[29,43,72]

GENERAL MOTOR ABILITY

General motor ability can be defined as the inherited and learned capacity demonstrated in the performance of fundamental skill activities.[38] Components such as muscular strength, muscular endurance, power, speed, cardiovascular endurance,

TABLE 6.1
General Motor Ability

1. **Component Structure**
   Muscular Strength
   Musclular Endurance
   Power
   Speed
   Cardiovascular Endurance
   Flexibility
   Agility
   Coordination
2. **Related to Athletic Classification**
3. **Transferability and Relatedness of Physical Activities**

TABLE 6.2

1. **Performance Related**
2. **Specific to Designated**
   Physical Activity Movement Parameters
3. **Little Transferability**
   Between Designated
   Physical Activity
   Movement Parameters

flexibility, agility, and coordination were established, and tests were developed as measures of these factors.[6,8,48,54,62] Measures of this type were aimed at the predictive evaluation of athletic performance and the homogenous classification of students for physical education classes.

Early research studies in this field of interest were conducted basically in the establishment of such components relative to their relatedness and transferability to athletic skill activity (Figure 6.1). Factor analysis statistical techniques were utilized to find these principal factors or components. Fleishman and Hempel,[17] in an investigation of complex motor performance, reported the generality of factor characteristics found in their results. The components identified as general were those of: coordination, spatial interpretations, direction discrimination ability, pursuit speed adjustment, visual comparison ability, and manipulation facility. Similarly, Ackerman[1] found motor ability to be related to speed and accuracy of given movement parameter foundations. Cumbee et al.[13] investigated the relatedness and nonrelatedness between components in their study of motor coordination. Their findings demonstrated a similarity between the balancing of objects and change of direction speed in relation to arm and hand movements, and dissimilarity between the components of total body change of direction and body balance.

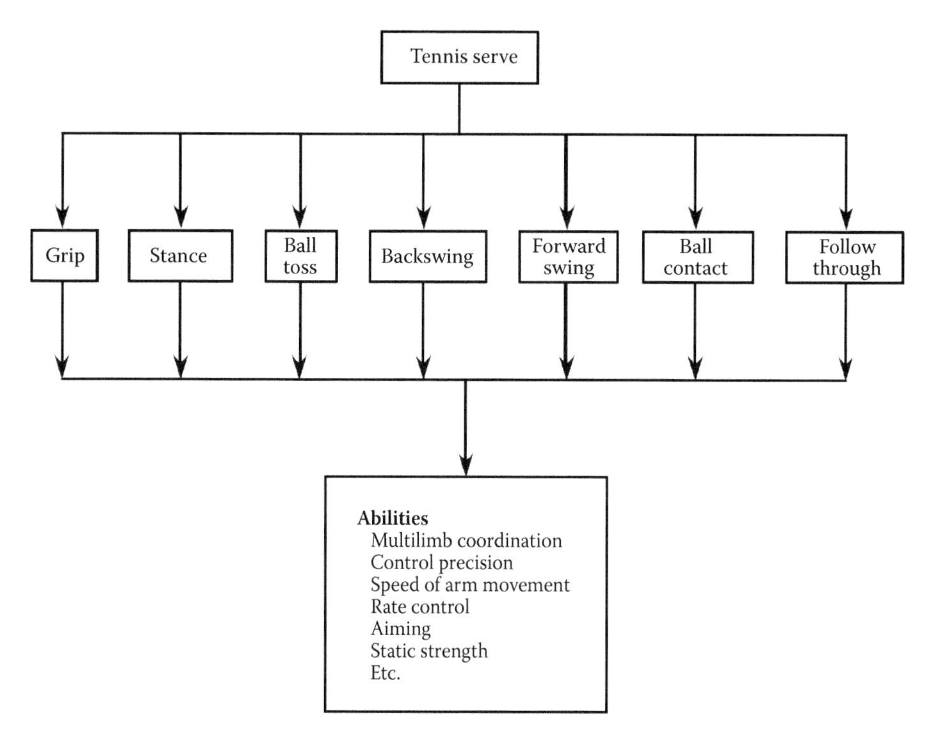

FIGURE 6.1 Underlying general motor abilities (tennis serve). (From Magill, R.A., *Motor Learning and Motor Control: Concepts and Applications,* 7th ed., McGraw-Hill, Boston, 2004. With the permission of the McGraw-Hill Companies.)

Subsequent research investigations in this area of study were more demonstrative of a general to specific ability of change relative to proficiency under practice conditions. Fleishman[20] found that such abilities were basically general in nature, resulting from movement consistencies in the performance of designated task activities. Safrit[57] studied heterogeneous skilled groups of subjects and found movement similarity in throwing, kicking, pushing, and striking factor skills. Her findings demonstrated that these factor similarities contributed to the performance levels achieved by the groups involved. Subsequent reports from studies such as those of Fleishman,[21,22] Fleishman and Rich,[21] Humphrey,[32] and Jones[33] were indicative of this change in that their findings revealed that, while motor abilities were general in the initial stages of learning, they became more specific with practice (Table 6.3).

Motor ability models were also developed in this area of study in order to functionally describe the nature and scope of such abilities relative to learning. Fleishman[20] formulated an ability to skill paradigm to show the general to specific process evident in motor learning. Fitts[16] classified motor ability and motor learning processes in terms of three categories or phases. The first phase was cognitive in nature and involved an understanding of the task to be learned. Phase two was associative and practice centered, and phase three was autonomous, wherein skilled levels of movement patterns were fully learned. Overlearning in this regard may be

TABLE 6.3
Generalized and Descriptive Patterns of Motor Learning

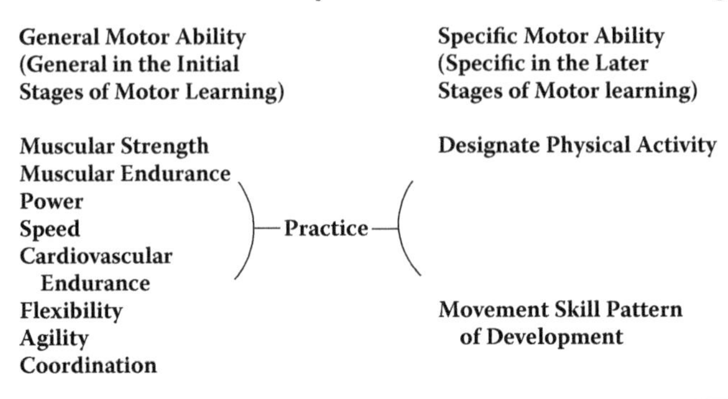

General Motor Ability (General in the Initial Stages of Motor Learning)		Specific Motor Ability (Specific in the Later Stages of Motor learning)
Muscular Strength		Designate Physical Activity
Muscular Endurance		
Power		
Speed	Practice	
Cardiovascular Endurance		
Flexibility		Movement Skill Pattern of Development
Agility		
Coordination		

advised to ensure an increase in autonomous levels of motor skill.[24] Cratty[12] established a three-level theory that described motor performance to include the parameters of general physical support behaviors, perceptual motor traits, and task-specific factors. Stallings[73,74] developed an instructional model which encompassed the state of the learner, the instructional methods utilized, and the nature of the task to be learned. She related these factors to preplanning and continuous change phases relative to motor development and proficiency levels. Similarly, Vereyker et al.[77] also proposed a learning model related to the learner/task dynamics of application. The inherent changes in this interaction of learner to task were linked to individual learning processes relative to task problem solving.

SPECIFIC MOTOR ABILITY

The predominance of research in motor ability has been advanced in support of specificity.[43] Seashore[63] basically established the specificity of motor ability. He found that fine and gross motor abilities were essentially independent, and that no general overall relationship existed between the two classifications. Fleishman[18,19] studied 24 static and movement motor ability tasks and found them to be specific in nature.[1] Studies such as these advanced the concept of specificity in the area of motor ability. Abilities were found to be nontransferable and related to the undertaken physical tasks. Henry and Rogers[29,30] were probably the prime movers of specificity in motor learning. They devised the memory drum theory, in which the brain was the repository for storage of neuromotor movement patterns which were utilized when afferent messages and efferent responses were to be made. Similarly, Lotter,[41] Bachman,[5] Cratty,[11] Smith,[72] Singer,[69] and Loockerman and Berger[40] found low correlations between cranking movements, ladder balance, adductor movement speed, throwing and kicking, and reactive directional movement times, respectively.

To date, the results of studies are demonstrable of continuing debatable positions. According to Magill,[43] little evidence has been reported in support of general motor abilities. In contrast, studies by Keele and Hawkins[35] and Keele et al.[36,37] suggest that there is some support for the existence of general motor abilities. Their correlation findings on movement, timing, and force control were indicative of ability similarities derived from partial related processes shared by different tasks. Landers et al.[39] corroborated their findings in their study on archery performance. Perceptual motor and psychological characteristics were found to be predictors of performance abilities.

MOTOR CONTROL

Motor movements are generally under the control of the cerebral cortex, the basal ganglia, and the cerebellum (Figure 6.2).[14,26,75] The cerebral cortex receives, interprets, sends out, and stores sensory information. The basal ganglia serve as a relay mechanism that can initiate and translate the motor program responses selected.[25] The refining process of motor skill patterning is in the control of the cerebellum. Here, the coordinative adjustments are made. These three systems form a relay loop unit that basically organizes and reorganizes the structural formation and reformation of planned motor movements.[47] The cerebellum, in concert with the brain stem, monitors descending signals in comparison to ascending feedback.[2,15,23,26] The brain stem also forms a relay circuit with the spinal cord in the coding of incoming and outgoing signals in the control process of voluntary and involuntary movements to be made.[43] From the spinal cord, the eventual motor neuron signals are transmitted

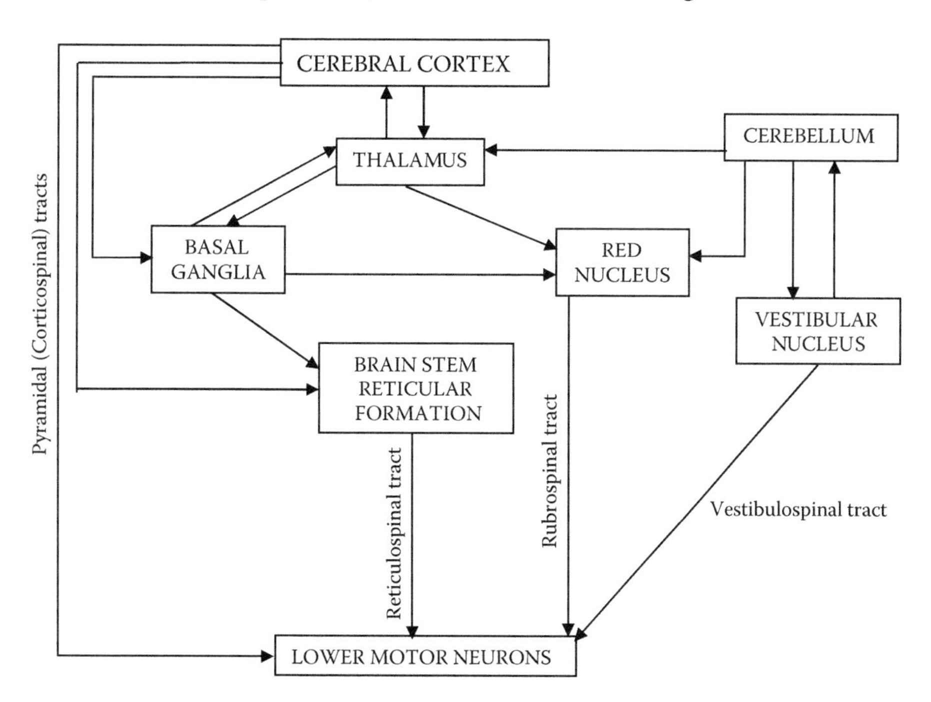

FIGURE 6.2 Centers and pathways of neural motor control of skeletal muscles. (From Fox, S.I., *Human Physiology,* 2nd ed., W.C. Brown Publishers, Dubuque, IA, 1987. Reproduced with the permission of the McGraw-Hill Companies.)

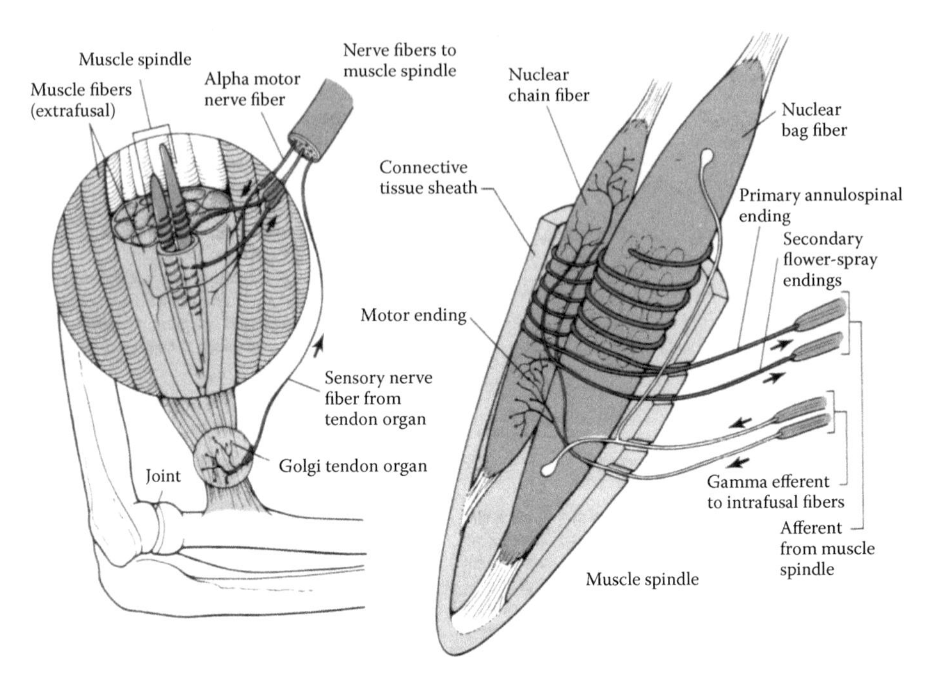

FIGURE 6.3 Structure and location of muscle spindles in skeletal muscle. (From Powers S.K. and T.T. Howley, *Exercise Physiology: Theory and Application to Fitness and Performance,* 2nd ed., Brown and Benchmark, Madison, WI, 1994. Reproduced with the permission of the McGraw-Hill Companies.)

to designated muscle groups for the motor responses selected for execution. Also involved in motor movement processes are the muscle spindles and Golgi tendon organs. These two systems govern the amount of stretch involved in the shortening and lengthening of muscle tissue during movement.[27,47,51,54,60,80] Muscle spindles found in the interior portion of muscle tissue facilitate contraction and stretch, while Golgi tendon organs located in the tendinous end of muscle tissue inhibit contraction and stretch to protect muscle tissue from possible injury (Figure 6.3).[51]

CLOSED AND OPEN LOOP MOTOR LEARNING

Parallel advances in motor learning research during this time in relation to closed (specific) and open (general) loop theories of motor movement have also been demonstrative of this controversy, but within different parameters. Poulton[52] described closed loop learning as skill performance governed by the self-regulation of neural adjustments relative to feedback processes, and open loop learning as the exemplification of skill performance bound to preplanned general sequences of movement phases made under changing situations and environments (Figure 6.4).

Two representative systems in this field of research were those formulated by Adams[2,3] and Schmidt.[59] Adams[2,3] described motor learning to be closed looped within the framework of memory and perceptual trace processes. Recall functions

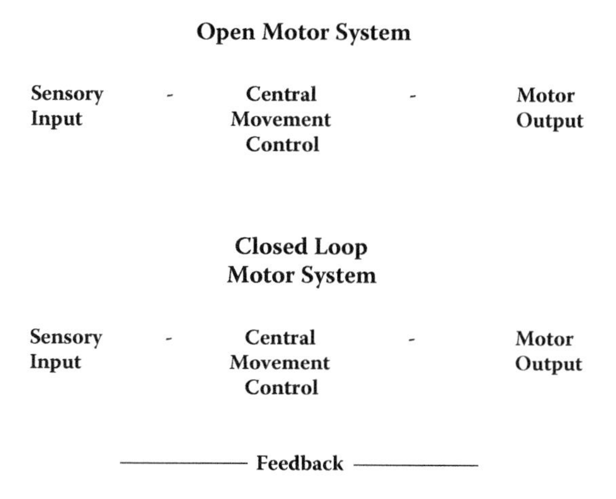

FIGURE 6.4 Open and closed loop motor learning systems.

in the selection and initiation of motor responses were under the control of memory traces, while perceptual traces served as the feedback response selection mechanism relative to recognition of previous movement patterns. Such trace-governed movements were specific, since they were based on selective neural and transmission operational functions. In contrast, Schmidt's schema theory[55,59,60] was open looped in nature and was set within the context of generalized motor planning movement conditions. Two schema plans are formed.[59,60] The first is the generalized motor program, which in essence controls the overall instructional phase of the activity to be learned (Figure 6.5). The second is the motor response component, which in turn relates the specifics of an action to the existing situation (Figure 6.6). The motor response program can be broken down into two parts, the recall schema and the recognition schema. The recall schema is accountable for the specific characteristics of the activity undertaken, and the recognition schema enables the learner to compare the actual to expected movement pattern outcomes and the adjustments to be made. Each skill activity to be learned is governed by:

1. Initial conditions — the movement patterns to be undertaken relative to the environmental existing context
2. Response specifications — the required specific activity characteristics of the skill to be performed
3. Sensory consequences — the sensory feedback after activity pattern is completed
4. Response outcome — the comparison of the actual performance to the expected results

CLOSED AND OPEN LOOP STUDIES

Studies in this area of research have encompassed the parameters of specificity and speed of feedback responses, and the generality and movement performance

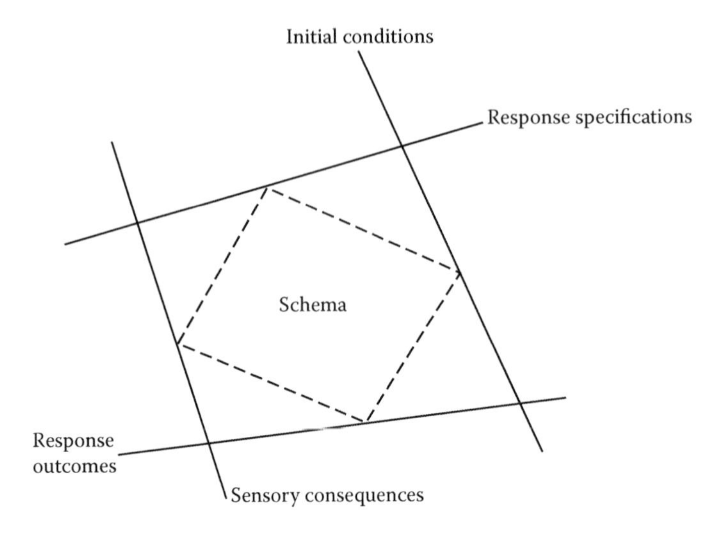

FIGURE 6.5 Generalized open loop motor learning schema. (From Kerr, R., *Psychomotor Learning,* Saunders College Publishing, New York, 1982. With the permission of the McGraw-Hill Companies.)

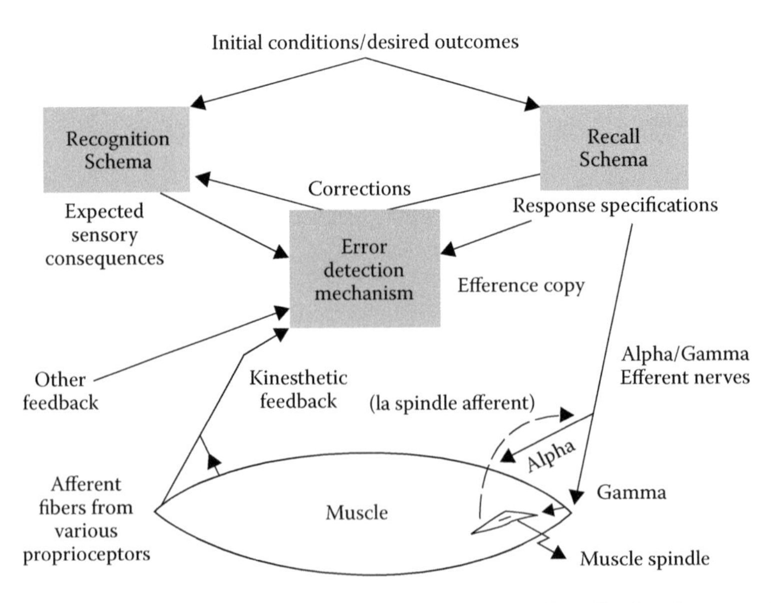

FIGURE 6.6 Schema theory motor response program. (From Kerr, R., *Psychomotor Learning,* Saunders College Publishing, New York, 1982. With the permission of the McGraw-Hill Companies.)

plans made in relation to different situations and conditions.[71] Howell[31] reported that immediate feedback in the learning of motor skills was essential for the identification and correction of wrong movement responses. Watkins[78] studied batting skills and found that television feedback was important to the learning of such movement patterns. Similarly, Gray and Brumbach,[28] in a study of badminton skills, found film loop feedback to be significant to skill acquisition. However, Sevennin et al.[64] later found general feedback to be better than kinematic feedback in the learning of different limb movements. In reference to the amount of feedback needed, Malina[45] found that throwing speed and accuracy were dependent upon the kind and completeness of feedback processes utilized. Winstein and Schmidt[81] reported that too much feedback could be of negative value relative to the learning process. Learners could become dependent upon the external cues given and negate their own sensory sources. These studies indicate that feedback must be immediate, related to type, complete, instructional, and processed in meaningful amounts. The basic limitation of closed loop systems is related to failure of sensory feedback processes to occur fast enough during quick movements. However, during slower and continuous movement patterns, feedback can be used more effectively in regard to flexible modifications of kinesthetic bodily motor control.[43,60,61]

In reference to open loop motor research studies, Saltz[58] found motor responses to be dependent upon existent characteristics set within internal and external conditions. Shapiro and Schmidt[65] reported that muscle contraction timing sequence phasing and the application of muscle forces were representative in the learning of movement pattern programs. Modification of these muscle forces becomes conditional to the motor skill task undertaken. Singer,[70] in his review of motor learning, found skill acquisition to be dependent upon both closed and open looped systems of learning. He concluded that, in the early phases of motor learning, previous motor experiences to selected kinds of movement patterns were significant, while in later phases motor responses became more specific because of operational feedback processes.[67] Margolis and Christina[46] utilized Schmidt's schema theory in their study of performance proficiency in target shooting. They found learning to be related to differences in practice situations and conditions during training. These studies indicate that advance instructional plans become essential to the learning of motor skills when:

1. The characteristics of given movement patterns make motor preprogramming necessary.
2. The sequencing of muscular forces become conditional to change.
3. The general quantitatives of movement lead to the specific qualitatives of movement.
4. The variabilities inherent in practice are situational and conditional.

The basic limitations of open loop systems are related to the significance of generalized variability of motor skill acquisition relative to specificity, and to the learning of new skills relative to motor control.[43,60,61]

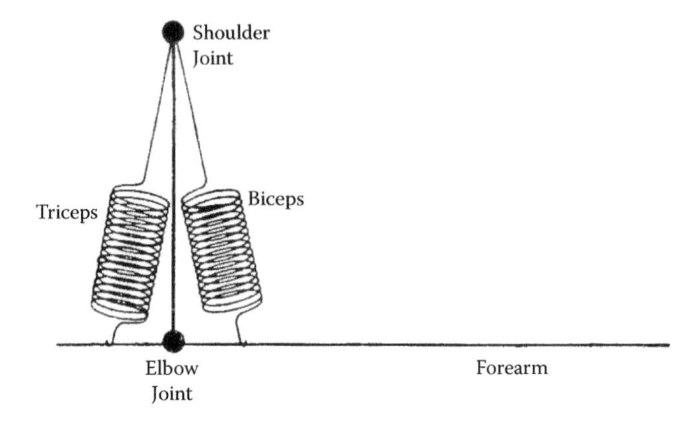

FIGURE 6.7 Dynamic systems theory model. (From Magill, R.A., *Motor Learning Concepts and Applications,* 4rth ed., Brown and Benchmark, Madison, WI, 1993. With the permission of the McGraw-Hill Companies.)

DYNAMIC AND EXPLORATORY MOTOR LEARNING APPROACHES

In contrast to open and closed looped motor learning theories are the dynamic and exploratory approaches to the learning of motor skills.[9,43,76] The dynamic systems theory is based on the functional pattern of coordinative muscle groups in movement that are synchronous and self organizational in nature (Figure 6.7). Agonistic and antagonistic muscle groups integratively work as reflexive units in movement relative to the stable constancy and unstable variability of active maintenance and changes in levels of physical activity. These changes occur in an autonomous manner as coordinative movement relationships in increasing and decreasing intensities are made relative to aerobic, anaerobic, and resistance training. The exploratory motor learning approach is process based on the coordinative integration of perception to action, bound by task and environmental limitations. Perceptive and active motor searches are made exploratively through workspace boundaries. These searches can provide the perceptual variables and feedback information to find optimal solutions to the learning of motor skills.

PRACTICE AND MOTOR LEARNING

In the acquisition of motor skill, practice plays a significant role. The application of practice variables essential to the learning process has been demonstrative of an increase in performance ability. The principles that have become prominent in this area of study have been centered in the following practice factors:[4,7,25,34,42,43,49,50,56,60,67,68,79,80,82]

1. Amount of time — The more time spent in practice, the greater the increase in motor skill.
2. Practice distribution — Massed practice or practice that involves short rest periods would be more effective for motor learning purposes than

distributed practice or practice with long rest periods in activities that are discrete in nature. In activities that are continuous, distributed practice would be more effective.

3. Whole/part practice — Whole method practice is better than part method practice when skills to be learned are low in complexity and high in organization. Part practice would be more effective when skills are high in complexity and low in organization.
4. Feedback — Information feedback can affect motor learning processes in a positive sense if it is administered at appropriate times and is specific in nature.
5. Overlearning — Practice beyond the normal amount of time spent in learning skills would be an effective methodology to employ, since the skills would become internalized.
6. Demonstration — Motor skills can be effectively learned through the use of modeling, wherein the skill to be learned can be operationally seen and then simulated.
7. Specificity — Motor skills can be effectively learned when simulated as closely as possible to the particular skill parameters of a given task.
8. Mental practice — Mental imagery and visual rehearsal of skills can be of positive value to the learning of skills.
9. Variable practice — The practice of one skill within different parameters of learning can increase the general application of that skill to performance.
10. Contextual interference — The practice of various skills during each training session can be of positive value in reference to the transfer of those skills to different performance parameters.

MOTOR ABILITY AND MOTOR LEARNING

While a summary of the research studies covered denotes the specificity of motor ability, its general nature cannot be negated. The theory and practice of motor ability study has demonstrated the progressive developments that have revised the earlier generality to the specificity of today relative to the underlying mechanisms indigenous to motor learning. The trends that have emerged from the research literature in this regard over the years indicate that motor ability acquisition through motor learning processes may be dependent upon general as well as specific factors. The general components of motor ability have become the practical quantitative physical supports to motor learning, while skill specificities have been demonstrated to be representative of neural processes and mechanisms exemplified in such learning. Similarly, closed and open loop study has shown that generality factors may be significant to motor learning in the earlier phases, while the specificity of feedback processes may be important to the later stages of performance learning. In retrospect, therefore, while motor ability study has been continued in the larger field of motor learning, the generality–specificity controversy is still evident within these different parameters of study. Added to these views are the dynamic and exploratory approaches to motor learning. They have been centered on functional and coordinative movement patterns responsive to exercise changes and perceptive activity processes related to given boundaries, respectively.

SUMMARY

In summary, the studies reviewed indicated that:

1. General motor ability is based on innate and acquired skill acquisition that is termed to be transferable in nature. Components such as those of muscular strength, muscular endurance, cardiovascular endurance, speed, power, agility, and coordination are utilized as the determinant factors. These component determinants should be used as the quantitative and underlying physical supports to motor learning. Resistance exercise conditioning programs designed for the development of these quantitative supports should be utilized.
2. Specific motor ability theory is based upon indigenous neural motor functions, the factors, and separate nontransferable skills. Qualitative plans should be formulated that are specifically and realistically designed for designated motor skill acquisition.
3. Motor movements are generally under the control of the cerebral cortex, the basal ganglia, and the cerebellum.
4. Closed loop motor learning is based upon self-regulating neural feedback from internal as well as external stimuli. Plans should be developed for the overlearning of designated skills to the point of automaticity under given situations and conditions.
5. Open loop motor learning is based upon the formulation of motor programs and the applicable variability of the motor factors involved. Practice plans should be developed that will ensure coverage of fundamental motor patterns to be learned. An understanding of the complexity and execution of such skills relative to the force factors involved is paramount to the formulation of motor plans.
6. Closed and open loop motor learning may be interactive in process relative to general motor programming in the beginning stages of learning and then become specific and feed back related in the later stages of motor acquisition. Practice plans should be formulated that will ensure such stages of learning in order that basic as well as advanced motor skills can be developed more fully.
7. Dynamic motor learning is based on the functional pattern of coordinative muscle groups in movement that are synchronous and self organizational in nature.
8. Exploratory motor learning is process based relative to the coordinative integration of perception to action, bound by task and environmental limitations
9. In the acquisition of motor skill, practice plays a significant role. The practice variables of time, distribution, whole/part learning, feedback,

overlearning, demonstration, specificity, and mental review must be operationally administered within appropriate instructional parameters.

GLOSSARY

Agility Rapid change of direction while in movement

Closed loop motor learning The learning of motor skills through the utilization of neural feedback information that would continually regulate action–reaction movement patterns to be made

Contextual interference The practice of different skills during individual training session that, in essence, interfere with one another relative to learning

Coordination Learned movement patterns that are the resultant of the integrated unity of singular skills

Demonstration The modeling of a motor skill through instructional performance procedures

Distributed practice Practice periods that include shorter sessions of activity and longer rest periods

Dynamic motor learning theory The functional pattern of coordinative muscle groups in movement that are synchronous and self organizational in nature

Exploratory motor learning theory The coordinative integration of perception to action bound by task and environmental limitations

Feedback Information transmitted to the brain that is related to movement pattern execution

Fine motor abilities Movement patterns that require the utilization of small muscle coordinative activity

Flexibility The extent to which a muscle or group of muscles can functionally move through a range of motion around a joint

General motor ability The general underlying capacity of an individual to perform a number of physical skills

Golgi tendon organs Sensory receptors that govern the stretching limits of muscular movement

Gross motor abilities Movement patterns that require the utilization of large muscle coordinative activity

Massed practice Practice periods that include short rest intervals between longer activity sessions

Memory drum theory The brain is the repository for the storage of neuromotor movement patterns that can be recalled when needed

Memory trace Recall functions in the selection and initiation of motor responses

Motor unit The neuron and the innervated muscle fibers involved in muscle contraction processes

Muscle spindles Intrafusal muscle fibers that are involved in the rate and amount of muscle stretch

Muscular endurance Submaximal repetitive or sustained muscular exertion force against a resistance

Muscular strength Maximal muscular exertion of force against resistance during one trial effort
Open loop motor learning The learning of motor skills through pre-planned program practice execution
Overlearning Practice that is extended beyond normal learning limits
Perceptual motor abilities A group of abilities that are involved in the execution of activities related to the speed and accuracy of movement
Perceptual trace Feedback response selection mechanisms relative to recognition of previous movement patterns
Power The amount of work performed per unit of time
Schema theory Subjective preplanned programs in the learning of motor skills
Specificity The practice summation of performance parameters, indigenous to the motor skill to be learned
Specific motor ability Abilities that are specific to the nature of the skill to be performed
Speed Rapidity in repeated patterns of movement
Stabilometer A piece of equipment that measures balance
Stamina The cardiovascular endurance that can be demonstrated during prolonged physical activity
Transfer The amount of skill acquired in a motor task that is related to the practice influence of another learned movement pattern
Variable practice Practice periods that include the learning of individual skills within different parameters of learning
Whole/part motor learning The learning of motor skills through complete trials or through designated segments

REFERENCES

1. Ackerman, P.L., Determinants of individual differences during skill acquisition. Cognitive abilities and information processing, *Journal of Experimental Psychology,* 117, 288–818, 1988.
2. Adams, J.A., A closed loop theory of motor behavior, *Journal of Motor Behavior,* 3, 111–149, 1971.
3. Adams, J.A., The changing face of motor learning, *Human Movement Science,* 9, 209–220, 1990.
4. Adams, W.C., *Foundations of Physical Education, Exercise and Sport Sciences,* Lea and Febiger, Philadelphia, 1991.
5. Bachman, J.C., Specificity vs. generality in learning and performing two large muscle motor tasks, *Research Quarterly,* 32, 3–31, March, 1961.
6. Beunen, G. and J. Borms, Kinanathropometry: roots, developments and future, *Journal of Sports Sciences,* 8, 1–15, 1990.
7. Christina, R.W. and R.A. Bjork, Optimizing long term retention and transfer, in *In the Minds Eye: Enhancing Human Performance,* Druckman, D. and R.A. Bjork, Eds., National Academy Press, Washington, DC, 1991.
8. Clarke, H.H., *Application of Measurement to Health and Physical Education,* Prentice-Hall, Englewood Cliffs, NJ, 1976.

9. Cook, A.S. and M.H. Woolacott, *Motor Control Through Practical Applications,* Williams and Wilkins, Baltimore, 1995.
10. Cozens, F.W., *The Measurement of General Athletic Ability in College Men,* University of Oregon Press, Eugene, OR, 1929.
11. Cratty, B.J., Effects of intra-maze delay upon learning, *Perpetual Motor Skills,* 15, 14, 1962.
12. Cratty, B.J., A three level theory of perceptual motor behavior, *Quest,* May, 1966.
13. Cumbee, F.Z., M. Meyer, and G. Peterson, Factorial analysis of motor coordination variables for third and fourth grade girls, *Research Quarterly,* 28, 100–108, May 1957.
14. Edington, D.W. and V.R. Edgerton, *The Biology of Physical Activity,* Prentice-Hall, Englewood Cliffs, NJ, 1976.
15. Fisher, A.G. and C.R. Jensen, *Scientific Basis of Athletic Conditioning,* 3rd ed., Lea and Febiger, Philadelphia, 1990.
16. Fitts, P.M, Perceptual-motor skill learning, in *Categories of Human Learning,* Melton, A.W., Ed., Academic Press, New York, 1964.
17. Fleishman, E.A. and W.E. Hempel, Jr., Factorial analysis of complex psychomotor performance and related skills, *Journal of Applied Psychology,* 40, 96–604, 1956.
18. Fleishman, E.A., A comparative study of aptitude patterns in unskilled and skilled psychomotor performances, *Journal of Applied Psychology,* 41, 263–372, 1957.
19. Fleishman, E.A., An analysis of positioning movements and static reactions, *Journal of Experimental Psychology,* 55, 13–34, 1958.
20. Fleishman, E.A., The description and prediction of perceptual motor skill learning, in *Training, Research, and Education,* Glaser, R., Ed., University of Pittsburgh Press, 1962, republished, John Wiley, New York, 1965.
21. Fleishman, E.A. and S. Rich, Role of kinesthetic and spatial visual abilities in perceptual motor learning, *Journal of Experimental Psychology,* 66, 6–61, 1963.
22. Fleishman, E.A., *The Structure and Measurement of Physical Fitness,* Prentice-Hall, Inc., Englewood Cliffs, NJ, 1964.
23. Fox, E.L., R.W. Bowers, and M.L. Foss, *The Physiological Basis for Exercise and Sport,* 5th ed., Brown and Benchmark, Madison, WI, 1993.
24. Gabbard, C.P., *Lifelong Motor Development,* Brown and Benchmark, Madison, WI, 1992.
25. Gensemer, R.E., *Physical Education: Perspectives, Inquiry, and Applications,* 3rd ed., Brown and Benchmark, Madison, WI, 1995.
26. Ghez, C. and J. Krakauer, The organization of movement, in *Principles of Neural Science,* 4th ed., Kandel, E.R., J.H. Swartz, and T.M. Jessell, Eds., McGraw-Hill Companies, New York, 2000.
27. Gordon, J. and C. Ghez, Muscle receptors and spinal reflexes: the stretch reflex, in *Principles of Neural Science,* 3rd ed., Kandel, E.R., J.H. Swartz, and T.M. Jessell, Eds., Appleton and Lange, Norwalk, CT, 1991.
28. Gray, C.A. and N.B. Brumbach, Effect of daylight projection of film loops on learning badminton, *Research Quarterly,* 38, 562–569, 1967.
29. Henry, F. and E. Rogers, Increased response latency for complicated movements and a memory drum theory of neuromotor reaction, *Research Quarterly,* 31, 449–957, October, 1960.
30. Henry, F., Reaction time-movement time correlations, *Perceptual and Motor Skills,* 12, 1962.
31. Howell, M.L., Use of force-time graphs for performance analysis in facilitating motor learning, *Research Quarterly,* 27, 12–22, 1956.

32. Humphrey, G., *Thinking: An Introduction to its Experimental Psychology,* Wiley and Sons, New York, 1963.
33. Jones, M.B., Individual differences, in *The Psychomotor Domain: Movement Behavior,* Singer, R.N., Ed., Lea and Febiger, Philadelphia, 1972.
34. Juaire, S. and D. Pargman, Pictures versus verbal instructions to assist the learning of a gross motor task, *Journal of Human Movement Studies,* 20, 189–900, 1991.
35. Keele, S.W. and H.L. Hawkins, Explorations of individual differences relevant to high level skill, *Journal of Motor Behavior,* 14, 3–33, 1982.
36. Keele, S.W., R.I. Ivory, and R.A. Pokorny, Force control and its relation to timing, *Journal of Motor Behavior,* 19, 96–614, 1987.
37. Keele, S.W. et al., Do perception and motor production share common timing mechanisms: a correlational analysis, *Acta Psychologica,* 60, 173–391, 1985.
38. Kerr, R., *Psychomotor Learning,* Saunders College Publishing, New York, 1982.
39. Landers, D.M., S.H. Boucher, and M.W. Wang, A psychobiological study of archery performance, *Research Quarterly for Exercise and Sport,* 57, 236–644, 1986.
40. Loockerman, W.D. and R.A. Berger, Specificity and generality between various directions for reaction and movement times under choice stimulus conditions, *Journal of Motor Behavior,* 4, 1972.
41. Lotter, W.S., Interrelationship among reaction times and speed of movement in different limbs, *Research Quarterly,* 31, 147–754, 1960.
42. Magill, R.A., Motor learning is meaningful for physical educators, *Quest,* 42, 126–633, 1990.
43. Magill, R.A., *Motor Learning and Control: Concepts and Applications,* 7th ed., McGraw-Hill Higher Education, New York, 2005.
44. Magill, R.A., Practice schedule considerations for enhancing human performance in sport, in *Enhancing Human Performance in Sport: New Concepts and Developments,* Christina, R.W. and H.M. Eckers, Human Kinetics, Champaign, IL, 1992.
45. Malina, R.M., Effects of varied information feedback practice conditions on throwing speed and accuracy, *Research Quarterly for Exercise and Sport,* 52, 474–483, 1981.
46. Margolis, J.F. and R.W. Christina, A test of Schmidt's schema theory of discrete motor skill learning, *Research Quarterly for Exercise and Sport,* 52, 474–483, 1981.
47. McArdle, W.D., F.I. Katch, and V.L. Katch, *Exercise Physiology: Energy, Nutrition, and Human Performance,* 3rd ed., Lea and Febiger, Philadelphia, 1991.
48. McCloy, C.H. and N.D. Young, *Tests and Measurements in Health and Physical Education,* Appleton-Century-Crofts, New York, 1954.
49. McCloy, C.H., *Tests and Measurements in Health and Physical Education,* F.S. Crofts and Co., New York, 1939.
50. Newell, K.M. and I. Rovegno, Commentary on motor learning: theory and practice, *Quest,* 42, 126–633, 1990.
51. Plowman, S.A. and D.L. Smith, *Exercise Physiology for Health, Fitness, and Performance,* 2nd ed., Benjamin Cummings, San Francisco, 2002.
52. Poulton, E.C., On prediction in skilled movements, *Psychological Bulletin,* 54, 467–778, 1957.
53. Robertson, S. and D. Elliott, Specificity of learning and dynamic balance, *Research Quarterly for Exercise and Sport,* 67, 69–95, 1996.
54. Rose, D.J., *A Multilevel Approach to the Study of Motor Control and Learning,* Allyn and Bacon, Boston, 1997.
55. Rosenbaum, D.A., *Human Motor Control,* Academic Press, San Diego, 1991.
56. Rudisill, M.E. and A.S. Jackson, *Theory and Application of Motor Learning,* Mac J.R. Publishing Company, Onalaska, TX, 1992.

57. Safrit, M.J., A study of selected object projection skills performed by subjects above average in skill, *Research Quarterly,* 40, 788–898, 1969.
58. Saltz, E., *The Cognitive Bases of Human Learning,* Dorsey Press, Homewood, IL, 1977.
59. Schmidt, R.A., A schema theory of discrete motor skill learning, *Psychological Review,* 82, 225–560, 1975.
60. Schmidt, R.A. and T.D. Lee, *Motor Control and Learning: A Behavioral Emphasis,* 4th ed., Human Kinetics Publisher, Champaign, IL, 2005.
61. Schmidt, R.A. and C. Wrisberg, *Motor Learning and Performance,* 3rd ed., Human Kinetics, Champaign, IL, 2004.
62. Scott, M.G., Motor ability tests for college women, *Research Quarterly,* 14, 402–405, December, 1943.
63. Seashore, H.G., Some relationships of fine and gross motor abilities, *Research Quarterly,* 13, 259–974, October, 1942.
64. Sevennin, S.P. et al., Acquiring bimanual skills, contrasting forms of information feedback for interlimb decoupling, *Journal of Experimental Psychology: Learning, Memory, and Cognition,* 19, 1328–8344, 1993.
65. Shapiro, D.C. and R.A. Schmidt, The schema theory: recent evidence and developmental implications, in *Psychomotor Learning,* Kerr, R., Ed., Saunders College Publishing, New York, 1982.
66. Shea, C.H. and D.L. Wright, *An Introduction to Human Movement, The Sciences of Physical Education,* Allyn and Bacon, Needham Heights, MA, 1997.
67. Shea, C.H., W.L. Shebilske, and I. Worchel, *Motor Learning and Control,* Prentice Hall, Englewood Cliffs, NJ, 1993.
68. Siedentop, D., *Introduction to Physical Education, Fitness and Sport,* Fifth ed., New York, McGraw-Hill Higher Education, 2004.
69. Singer, R.N., Comparison of inter-limb skill achievement in performing a motor skill, *Research Quarterly,* 27, 405–510, 1966.
70. Singer, R.N., *Motor Learning and Human Performance: An Application to Motor Skills and Movement Behaviors,* 3rd ed., Macmillan Publishing Co., New York, 1980.
71. Smith, K.U., The geometry of human motion and its' neural formulations, *American Journal of Physical Medicine,* 40, 1961.
72. Smith, L.E., Influence of neuromotor program alteration on the speed of a standard arm movement, *Perpetual and Motor Skills,* 15, 327–790, 1962.
73. Stallings, L.M., *Motor Learning: From Theory to Practice,* C.V. Mosby Co., St. Louis, 1982.
74. Stallings, L.M., *Motor Skills: Development and Learning,* Wm. C. Brown Publishers, Dubuque, IA, 1973.
75. Teasdale, N. et al., Determining movement onsets from temporal series, *Journal of Motor Behavior,* 25, 97–706, 1993.
76. Turvey, M.T., Coordination, *American Psychologist,* 45, 938–853, 1990.
77. Vereyker, B. et al., Free(z)ing degrees of freedom in skill acquisition, *Journal of Motor Behavior,* 24, 132–242, 1992.
78. Watkins, D.L., Motion pictures as an aid in correcting baseball batting faults, *Research Quarterly,* 34, 228–833, 1968.
79. Weinberg, R.S. and D. Gould, *Foundations of Sport and Exercise Psychology,* Human Kinetics, Champaign, IL, 1995.
80. Wilmore, J.H. and D.L. Costill, *Physiology of Sport and Exercise,* Human Kinetics, Champaign, IL, 1994.

81. Winstein, C.J. and R.A. Schmidt, Reduced frequency of knowledge of results enhances motor skill learning, *Journal of Experimental Psychology: Learning, Memory, and Cognition,* 16, 677–791, 1990.
82. Wuest, D.A. and C.A. Bucher, *Foundations of Physical Education* Exercise Science *and Sport,* 14th ed., McGraw-Hill Higher Education, New York, 2003.

7 Fatigue and Physical Performance

INTRODUCTION

The study of fatigue in reference to physical performance has been substantially investigated. Fatigue has been generally described as the physical tiredness and exhaustion that results from work and can also be characterized by diminished and erratic patterns of movement. In a formal sense, fatigue has been defined as a decrease in the production of force and a failure to continue constant exercise intensity levels.[5,40] Most of the research on fatigue has been centered within the physiological and psychological parameters of exercise and motor learning (Figure 7.1).

FATIGUE AND PHYSICAL PERFORMANCE: PAST PERSPECTIVES

Strength, aerobic, and anaerobic studies have demonstrated the relationship of short-term maximal and long-term submaximal work performance to the onset of increasing fatigue and exhaustion. Much of the early physiological research on the analysis of localized muscular strength and fatigue was through isometric and isokinetic testing. Clarke et al.,[9] using cable tension testing to study strength decrement, found that fatigue index patterns were not the same under different workload conditions. Kroll[28] obtained similar results in his research on isometric patterns of fatigue in female subjects divided into low, moderate, and high strength-level groups. The greatest strength losses were exhibited by the high strength group.[28] Clarkson et al.[10] corroborated these findings in their study on isokinetic fatigue patterns. In separate trial studies, their results indicated that the stronger subjects became exhausted at a faster rate. In reference to male and female strength levels, Clarke[8] found that, while strength decrement losses were greater for men than they were for women, men tired more slowly.

Fatigue patterns in slow- and fast-twitch muscle fibers were also studied. Thorstensson and Karlsson[54] found fast-twitch muscle fiber fatigue to be significantly related to isokinetic force decrease. Nilsson et al.[39] reported similar results in their study on muscle strength and fiber types. In a study designed to induce slow and fast rates of fatigue in power and endurance athletes through isometric testing, Kroll et al.[29] found the power-trained athletes to tire faster than the endurance-trained athletes. These results, however, were dissimilar to those obtained by Clarkson et

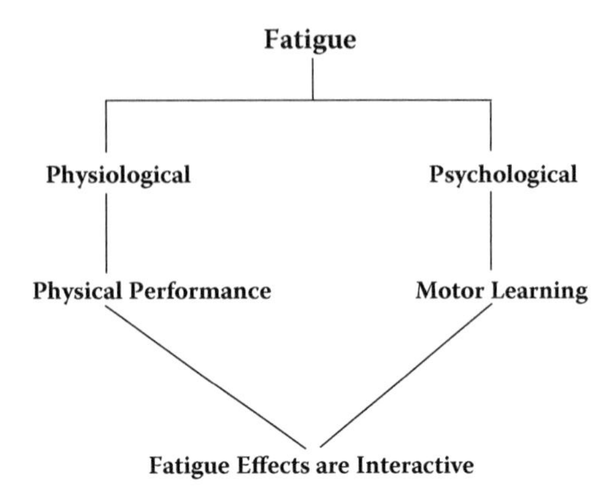

FIGURE 7.1 Fatigue related areas of study.

al.[10] They found muscle fiber composition to be unrelated to the decline of peak torque in college men tested through serial isokinetic strength procedures. These results were also corroborated by Thorstensson,[55] who found little relationship between fast-twitch muscle fibers and maximum isometric strength patterns. While these research results were contradictory in nature, Kroll[30] believed that the stronger relationship of isometric strength to muscle fiber composition may have influenced the obtained findings.

General and total body studies on fatigue relative to physical performance were centered in the areas of aerobic and anaerobic exercise processes. In reference to aerobic exercise, fatigue developed slowly (Figure 7.2).[57,59,62] Edwards[15] reported that fatigue resulting from aerobic work could well be due to calcium ion depletion. Nadel[36] found fatigue to be the result of glycogen depletion in the slow-twitch muscle fibers in his review of the cardiovascular adaptations to aerobic endurance training. McArdle et al.[34] attributed the glycogen depletion to an enzymatic failure in the transference of glycogen between the involved muscle tissues.

Anaerobic-induced fatigue relative to physical performance occurred quickly (Figure 7.3, Figure 7.4, Figure 7.5).[57] Davis,[12] in his anaerobic threshold study, found that during intensive work, the quick decrease in muscle and blood pH decreased glycolytic function and resulted in the fast onset of fatigue. Noakes[40] related anaerobic fatigue to the severe depletion of phosphocreatine stores. In a similar study, Davis[13] also reported that phosphocreatine depletion was the cause of anaerobic fatigue and that such depletion could well be the limiting factor to maximal intensive short-term performance. Lactic acid accumulation has also been related to anaerobic-induced fatigue. During intensive physical work, lactic acid increased in a corresponding manner to fatigue level; such production was said to be a precursor to the subsequent conditions that result and ultimately lead to severe exhaustion. These conditions include tissue acidity, calcium ion decrease, muscle tissue pH decrease, hydrogen ion accumulation, and contractile enzymatic inhibition.[20,27,36,40,43–45,62]

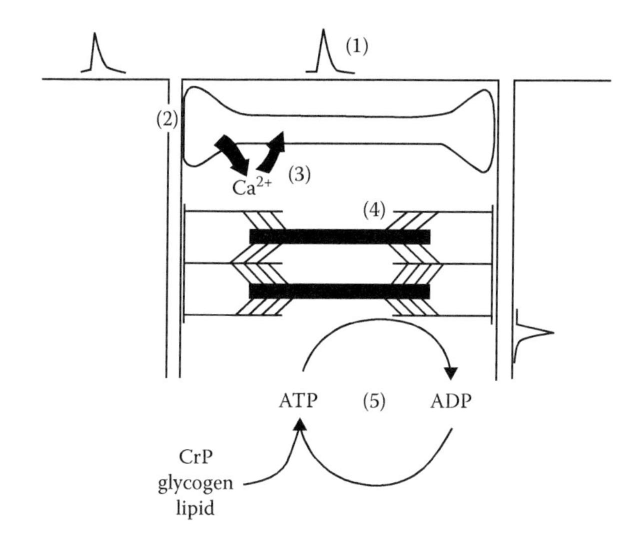

FIGURE 7.2 Possible sites and mechanisms of fatigue. 1. Action potentials — sarcolemma and T-tubules. 2. Transmission — T-tubules to SR membrane. 3. Calcium — release and reuptake. 4. Crossbridge formation. 5. ATP resynthesis. (From Vollestad, N.K. and O.M. Sejersted, *European Journal of Applied Physiology,* 57, 336–347, 1988. Copyright of Springer –Verlag. With the permission of the publisher.)

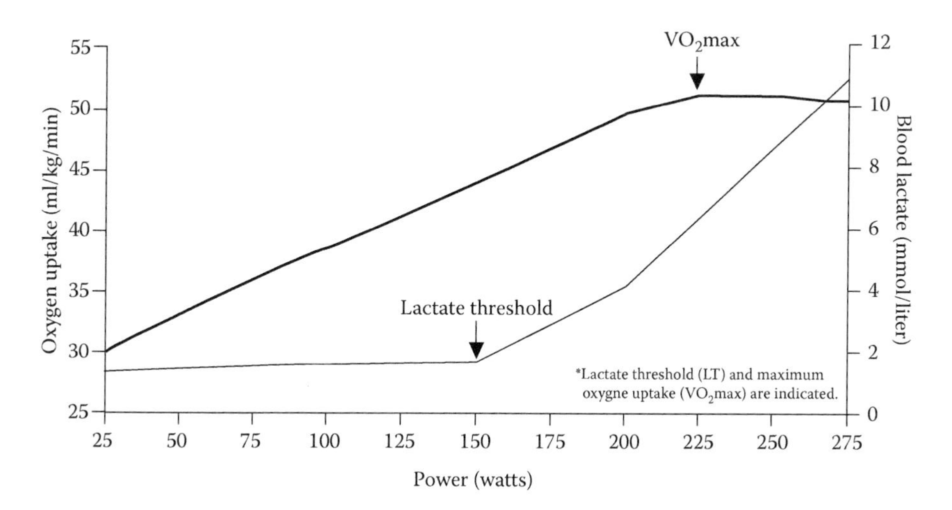

FIGURE 7.3 Oxygen uptake and blood lactate changes during increasing rates of cycle ergometer work. (From Physical Activity and Health: A Report of the Surgeon General. United States Department of Health and Human Services, 1996. With permission.)

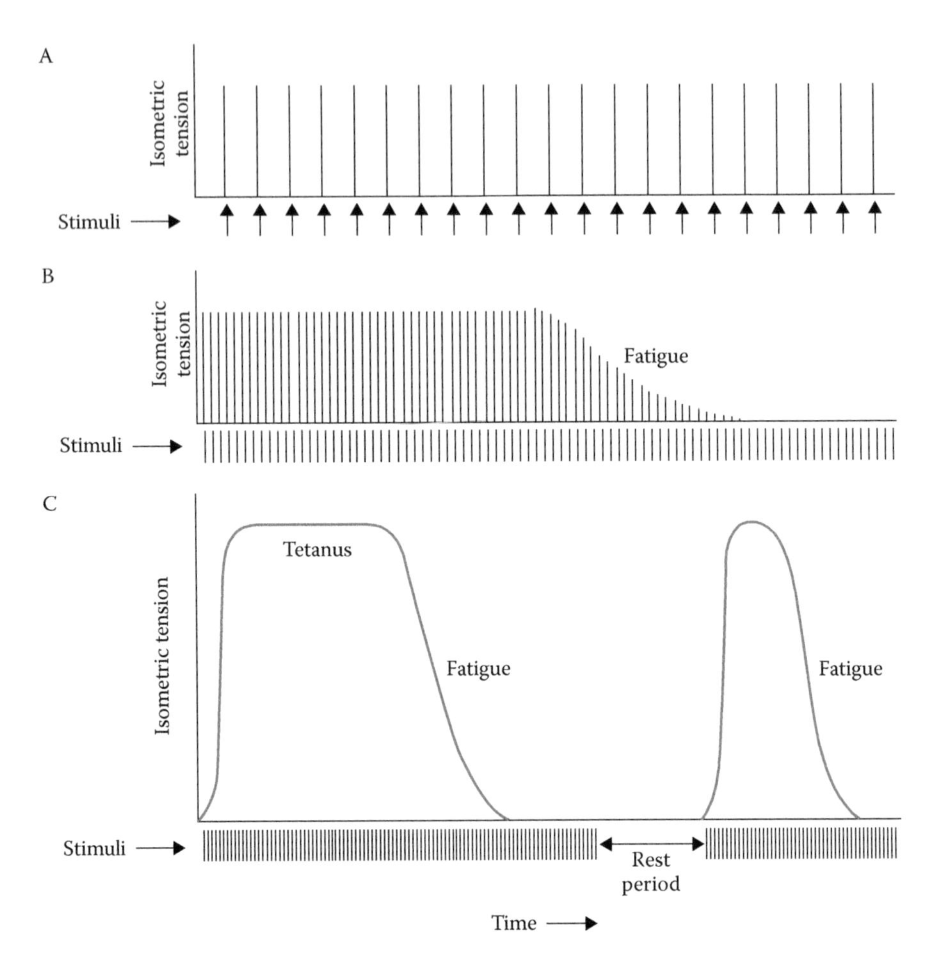

FIGURE 7.4 Muscular fatigue during (A) low-frequency twitch contractions, (B) high-frequency repeated twitch contractions, (C) maintained tetanus and recovery after rest period. (From Vander, A.J., J.H. Sherman, and D.S. Luciano, *Human Physiology: The Mechanisms of Body Function,* McGraw-Hill Publishing Company, New York, 1990. Reproduced with permission of the McGraw-Hill Companies.)

CURRENT PHYSIOLOGICAL CAUSES OF FATIGUE

Physiological research on the causes of fatigue due to exercise has been ongoing. The results of the research to date have been varied and somewhat complex. Recent research has been generally centered in central and peripheral neuromuscular system sites and mechanistic processes (Figure 7.6). Central nervous system failure, neural and muscular functions, and substrate depletion relative to fatigue have all been advanced as possible causes of exercise work decline.[2,3,11,12,14,16–18,20,22,25,28,32,40,41,43,46,53,57,63]

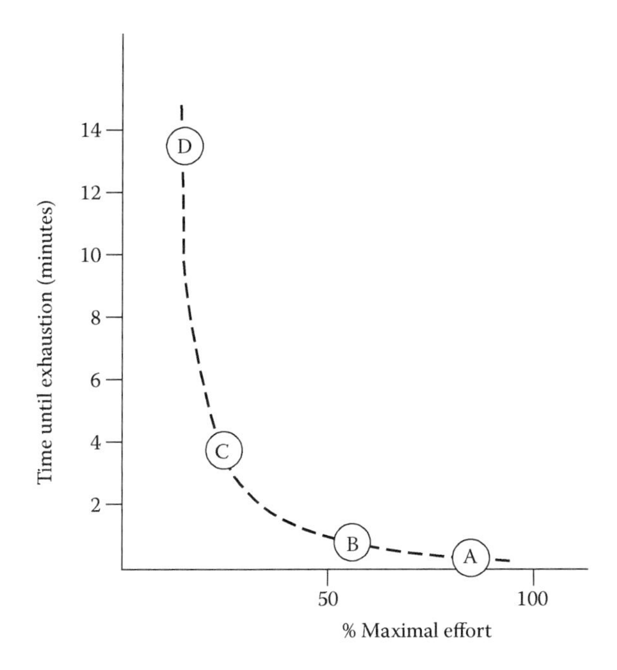

Key to graph	Running Distance	Time	Energy Source % Aerobic	% Anaerobic
A	100 m	10 sec	10	90
B	400 m	45 sec	25	75
C	1,500 m	3 min, 35 sec	55	45
D	5,000 m	13 min, 30 sec	85	15

FIGURE 7.5 Endurance exhaustion time for exercises performed at various aerobic and anaerobic levels. (From Wilmore, J.H. and J.A. Bergfeld, in *Sports Medicine and Physiology*, Strauss, R.H., Ed., W.B. Saunders, Philadelphia, 1979. With permission of the McGraw-Hill Companies.)

CENTRAL NERVOUS SYSTEM FATIGUE

Central nervous system failure relative to fatiguing work onset is related to the sensory signal and motor response transmission to and from the brain. Early studies by Merton[35] and Asmussen and Mazin[2] indicated that possibly failure to continue work was more psychologically than physiologically oriented.[43,57,62] The study by Merton[35] was related to electrical stimulation during exercise and increasing levels of fatigue. Muscle force decline continued, indicating that the central nervous system was not the causative factor.[33] In contrast, the study by Asmussen and Mazin[2] contended that, when diverting activities were used during weight training exercises and increasing fatigue, participants were able to continue work for longer periods of time. These results were indicative of some central nervous system influence over

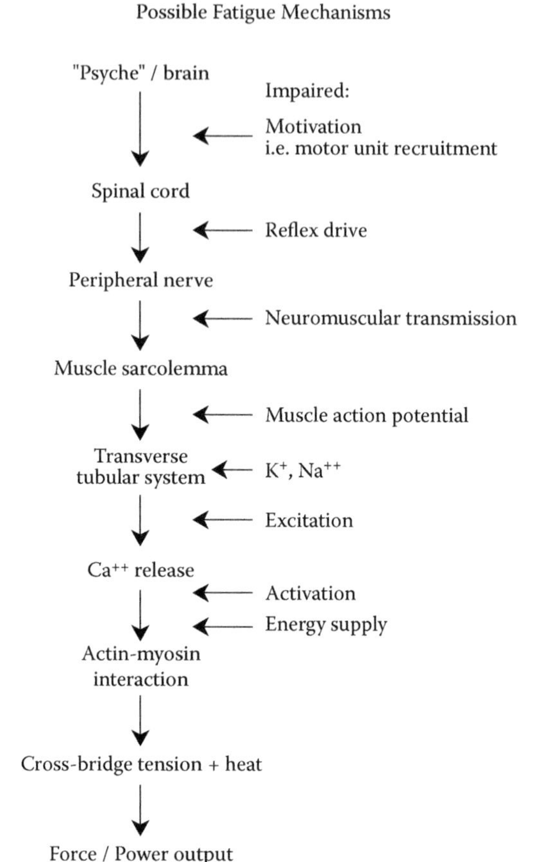

FIGURE 7.6 Fatigue sites and mechanisms. (From Powers S.K. and E.T. Howley, *Exercise Physiology: Theory and Application to Fitness and Performance,* 2nd ed., Brown and Benchmark, Madison, WI, 1994. With permission from the McGraw-Hill Companies.)

fatigue development.[43,61] Wilmore and Costill,[62] in their review of studies, indicate that fatigue onset may be used as a protective mechanism by the brain and that psychological encouragement may divert the feelings of exhaustion.

The role of amino acids in central nervous system failure has also been studied relative to the oxidation of the branched-chain amino acids (valine, leucine, and isoleucine) and tryptophan.[24,26] The supplementation of branched-chain amino acids has theoretically been reported to increase endurance levels.[52] In contrast, the intake of tryptophan, which is converted to serotonin (a neurotransmitter), has been related to a rise in fatigue.[37,41] During exercise, both the branched-chain amino acids and tryptophan compete for entry into the blood–brain barrier. When blood levels of branched-chain amino acids are high, theoretically the onset of fatigue is delayed. However, when this ratio is reversed, high tryptophan levels result in the increased production of serotonin, which in essence brings on fatigue more rapidly. In this regard, contrasting studies have been reported. Vandervalle et al.[58] studied glycogen-depleted participants in cycle ergometer exercise to exhaustion. No significant differences were found between the subjects taking branched-chain amino acid supplements and those in the control group. Segura and Ventura[48] in a study on tryptophan given to participants in 300-mg doses over a 24-h period resulted in an increased treadmill running time relative to perceived exertion ratings before fatigue and exhaustion set in. In contrast, Newsholme[37,38,54] believes tryptophan to be related to the onset of fatigue. The results of his studies are suggestive in this regard. He believes that, during endurance activities, branched-chain amino acid levels are decreased in the latter stages of the activity, allowing a greater amount of tryptophan to pass through the blood–brain barrier, resulting in a rise in serotonin levels and, subsequently, in increased rate of fatigue. Brouns,[6] in his review of amino acid–related fatigue, feels that further research is needed before theoretical substantiation can be made and reported. Recent research has also been related to the intake of carbohydrates which may normalize fatigue onset in this regard.[41,61,64]

PERIPHERAL NEUROMUSCULAR FATIGUE

Peripheral fatigue is generally related to neuromuscular transmission and substrate depletion processes. Transmission fatigue in this frame of reference can be the result of acetylcholine diffusion depletion at neuromuscular junction sites.[43,61] Fatigue may also be attributed to reduction of the action potential transmission in the sarcolemma and transverse tubules, indicating a possible decreased level of potassium and a reduced secretion of calcium ions (Figure 7.7).[19,21,34,43,61,62] These conditional effects can be demonstrated during maximal exercise levels when all of the motor units are firing and working. Electromyogram recordings at this time are indicative of reduced neural activity at the aforementioned sites.[34]

Substrate depletion

ATP

Phosphocreatine

Muscle glycogen

Blood-borne glucose

Metabolic by-products

Magnesium ions (Mg^{2+})

Adenosine diphosphate (ADP)

Inorganic phosphate (P_i)

Lactate ions

Hydrogen ions (H^+)

Ammonia

Reactive oxygen species

Heat

FIGURE 7.7 Metabolic factors in fatigue. (From Hargreaves, M., Metabolic factors in fatigue, Sports Science Exchange, Gatorade Sport Science Institute, 18, No. 3, 2005. With permission.)

Substrate-depletion fatigue is related to the exercise demands made on the body (Figure 7.6). This kind of fatigue is determined by muscle fiber type and short-term maximal and long-term submaximal work.[57] The firing rate of fast-twitch and slow-twitch muscle fibers differs. Fast-twitch muscle fibers are fast contracting, produce more lactic acid, and therefore fatigue faster than do the slow-twitch fibers, which contract slowly and produce lesser amounts of lactic acid. In short-term maximal exercise, fast-twitch muscle fibers predominate, but are also joined by an interaction of the slow-twitch fibers as all of the motor units become involved. There is an increase in lactic acid and metabolic end products. The rise in lactic acid is related to a rise in intracellular acidity and ammonia, an increase in hydrogen ion accumulation, and a decrease in calcium ion release that subsequently affect contractile mechanism processes, actin–myosin cross bridge binding, and the generation of muscular force.[17,32,34,43,53,57] There is also an accompanying decrease in muscle glycogen levels.[23,49] During long-duration submaximal work, slow-twitch muscle fibers predominate. Fatigue is related to a primary decrease in the glycogen levels of the slow-twitch fibers.[57] As glycogen levels are depleted, fast-twitch muscle fibers are recruited for use. When this occurs, the aforementioned fatigue effects that are set in motion during the onset of short-term intense work increase. There is also a decrease in adenosine triphosphate, creatine phosphate, and glucose levels.[24,53,57] The depletion of these substrates is related to a decrease in the exhitation and physical performance n-contraction coupling.[21]

Fatigue can also be caused by the bodily production of heat during exercise.[14,24,41,51,56] Both central and peripheral systems may be affected and, as a result, impair both short-intensive and long-endurance work through diminished muscle force generation.

FATIGUE AND MOTOR LEARNING

Psychological research has been related to the effects of fatigue on the learning of physical skills. Generally, studies have shown that, while fatigue affected physical performance, motor learning organismic function continued.[34,50] The research results, however, have been contradictory. Alderman[1] in his study on fatigue and training generalization for speed and accuracy, found that the learning of physical skills was not affected. Benson,[4] however, reported that learning relative to fatigue was related to the nature of the task. While speed was impaired in jumping, accuracy was enhanced in juggling after fatigue-induced bicycle ergometer work. Contrary to these findings, Pack et al.[42] found extreme fatigue to have a negative effect on motor learning. Treadmill-induced fatigue impaired learning processes on Bachman ladder trials.

Some psychological findings on fatigue and learning have also been related to fatigue offset through the utilization of motor-coordinative pattern movement changes.[31] Welford,[60] in his study on industrial fatigue, reported that, when work performance was affected by fatigue onset in a physiological manner, different patterns of movements were found to psychologically offset fatigue levels. The workload was then transferred over a larger body mass, resulting in a reduction of overall fatigue. These results were later corroborated by Bates et al.[3] and Elliot and

Ackland.[16] Running-induced fatigue in the late stages of road racing was offset by stride length, stride rate, body position, and speed changes.

Fatigue has also been related to practice methodology. During massed practices (long and intensive sessions), motor learning was negatively affected by fatigue onset, whereas during distributed practice (short and frequent sessions), motor learning was not influenced.[33] This may be due to the number and length of rest period intervals used during practice scheduling. Massed practices generally contain fewer and shorter rest periods, while distributed practices utilize longer and a greater number of rest sessions.

From the results of these representative studies, it is evident that fatigue is a conditional variable relative to motor learning. In a review of the literature, the fatigue effects on motor learning were found to be to be related to: [7,33,47]

1. Degree. Induced incremental levels of fatigue have a decremental effect on motor learning.
2. Point in time fatigue is induced. Earlier inducement of fatigue relative to the task to be learned results in a greater decremental effect on learning than would a later application of this conditional state.
3. Task dependency. Fatigue may be specific in its effect on motor learning.
4. Maintenance duration of fatigue application. Increased fatigue inducement time is incrementally related to learning decrement.

SUMMARY

In summary, these studies indicate that:

1. Fatigue has been defined as a decrease in the production of force and a failure to continue constant exercise intensity levels.
2. Central nervous system failure and neuromuscular transmission have been reported to be the physiological causes of fatigue. Fadeaway, substrate depletion, and amino acid–related fatigue have been reported to be the physiological causes of fatigue.
3. Central nervous system failure is related to sensory signal and motor response transmission to and from the brain.
4. Neuromuscular transmission fatigue can result from acetylcholine diffusion depletion at neuromuscular junction sites and from a reduction of the action potential transmission in the sarcolemma and transverse tubules.
5. Substrate depletion fatigue is related to the exercise demands made on the body. This kind of fatigue is determined by muscle fiber type and short-term maximal and long-term submaximal work.
6. Long-term submaximal fatigue is related to a depletion of glycogen in the slow-twitch muscle fiber types.
7. Short-term maximal induced fatigue is related to metabolic and causative processes in the fast-twitch muscle fiber types.
8. Amino acid–related fatigue has been related to the oxidation of the branched-chain amino acids and tryptophan.

9. Strength, anaerobic, and aerobic studies have demonstrated the relationship of short-term maximal and long-term submaximal work performance to the onset of increasing fatigue and exhaustion.
10. Isometric fatigue curve patterns differ when induced through different work resistance conditions.
11. Isometric fatigue curve patterns are different for similar workload conditions in reference to initial strength levels.
12. Even though men fatigue at slower rates than women, they demonstrate higher strength decrement levels.
13. Demonstrated isokinetic patterns of fatigue may be related to muscle fiber composition.
14. Power training programs induce faster rates of fatigue than do endurance training regimens.
15. Increasing fatigue levels are related to decreasing decrements in physical performance.
16. The effects of exercise-induced fatigue upon motor skill learning may be specifically related to the nature of the task.
17. Running-induced fatigue results in changes in movement patterns to promote performance time.
18. During massed practices (long and intensive sessions), motor learning can be negatively affected by fatigue onset, whereas during distributed practice (short and frequent sessions), motor learning may not be influenced.[33]
19. Fatigue effects on motor learning are related to degree, the point in time fatigue is induced, task dependency, and maintenance duration of fatigue application.
20. The onset of fatigue can be delayed through utilization of general and specific training programs.
21. Fast- and slow-twitch muscle fiber types can be metabolically optimized through specific utilization of distance, interval, and speed play training practices.
22. The learning of physical skills can be related to optimal time periods of practice relative to fatigue effects.
23. Alternate movement patterns can be designed to offset the fatigue effects of exercise.

GLOSSARY

Acetylcholine Chemical substance involved in neural impulse transmission

Action potential The electrical activity generated in the process of depolarization in nerve and muscle tissue

Adenosine triphosphate/creatine phosphate Immediate energy compound sources involved in muscle contraction processes

Aerobic Physical work done in the presence of oxygen

Amino acid–related fatigue The relationship of branched-chain amino acids and tryptophan to the onset of fatigue and subsequent exhaustion

Anaerobic Physical work done without the presence of oxygen

Branched-chain amino acids Amino acids that compete with tryptophan for entrance through blood brain barrier and are related to performance and the delay of fatigue onset

Central nervous system failure Sensory signal and motor response transmission to and from the brain regarding the decline of continuous fatiguing work

Distributed practice Short and frequent practice sessions

Fast-twitch fibers Muscle fibers that are anaerobic, fast contracting, and fast fatiguing

Fatigue Decrease in the production of force and a failure to continue constant exercise intensity levels

Glycogen The stored form of glucose in muscle and liver tissue

Isokinetic Refers to exercises that are executed at a constant speed throughout a full range of movement against an equal designated resistance

Isometric Refers to exercise that is nonmoving at given body angles for short periods of time against an immovable resistance

Lactic acid Anaerobic end product of glucose conversion to lactate

Massed practices Long and intensive practice sessions

Muscular strength and fatigue pattern curves Isometric and isokinetic measures of muscular strength decrease relative to the gradation of increasing fatigue levels

Neuromuscular junctions Axon/dendrite synapses

Neuromuscular transmission–reduced secretion of calcium Fatigue depletion of acetylcholine at neuromuscular junctions and at motor end plates. There may also be a reduction of the action potential transmission in the sarcolemma and transverse tubules, indicating a possible depletion of potassium and a calcium ions, respectively

pH level The acidity/alkalinity ratio levels in body fluids

Sarcolemma Membranous muscle tissue that covers individual muscle fibers

Serotonin A neurotransmitter involved in amino acid–related fatigue

Slow-twitch fibers Muscle fibers that are aerobic, slow contracting, and slow fatiguing

Substrate-depletion fatigue level During short-term maximal work, fast-twitch muscle fibers predominate, and as a result there is a rise in lactic acid and metabolic end products During long-term submaximal work, slow-twitch muscle fibers predominate, and as a result there is a decrease in gycogen, adenosine triphosphate, creatine phosphate, and glucose levels.

Transverse tubules Pathways through which neural impulses are conducted in order to activate calcium ions stored in sarcoplasmic reticulum

Tryptophan An amino acid related to an increase in fatigue levels when it passes through the blood–brain barrier and results in an increased level of serotonin

REFERENCES

1. Alderman, R.B., Influence of local fatigue on speed and accuracy in motor learning, *Research Quarterly,* 36, 131–140, 1965.
2. Asmussen, E. and B. Mazin, A central nervous component in local muscular fatigue, *European Journal of Applied Physiology,* 38, 9–15, 1978.
3. Bates, B.T., L.R. Osternig, and S.L. James, Fatigue effects in running, *Journal of Motor Behavior,* 9, 203–207, 1977.
4. Benson, D.W., Influence of imposed fatigue on learning a jumping task and juggling task, *Research Quarterly,* 39, 251–257, 1968.
5. Birch, K., D. MacLaren, and K. George, *Instant Notes: Sport and Exercise Physiology,* Garland Science/BIOS Scientific Publishers, London, 2005.
6. Brouns F. and C. Cargill, *Essentials of Sports Nutrition,* 2nd ed., John Wiley and Sons, New York, 2002.
7. Chamberlin, C. and T. Lee, Arranging practice conditions and designing instruction, in *Handbook of Research on Sport Psychology,* Singer, R.N., M. Murphy, and L.K. Tennant, Eds., Macmillan Publishing Company, New York, 1993.
8. Clarke, D.H., Sex differences in strength and fatigability, *Research Quarterly for Exercise and Sport,* 57, 144–149, 1986.
9. Clarke, D.H., C.T. Shay, and D.K. Mathews, Strength decrement index: a new test of muscle fatigue, *Archives of Physical Medicine and Rehabilitation,* 36, 368–376, 1955.
10. Clarkson, P.M. et al., The relationships among isokinetic endurance, initial strength level and fiber type, *Research Quarterly for Exercise and Sport,* 53, 15–19, 1982.
11. Conley, M., Bioenergetics of exercise and training, in *Essentials of Strength Training,* 2nd ed., Baechle, T.R. and R.W. Earle, Eds., Human Kinetics, Champaign, IL, 2000.
12. Davis, J.A., Anaerobic threshold: review of the concept and directions for future research, *Medicine and Science in Sports and Exercise,* 17, 6, 1985.
13. Davis, J.A., Response to Brook's manuscript, *Medicine and Science in Sports and Exercise,* 17, 32, 1985.
14. Drust, B. et al., Elevations in core and muscle temperature impair repeated sprint performance, *Acta Physiologica Scandinavica,* 183, 181–190, 2005.
15. Edwards, R.H.T., Human muscle function and fatigue, in *Human Muscle Fatigue: Physiological Mechanisms,* Ciba Foundation Symposium, Pitman Medical, London, 1981.
16. Elliot, B. and T. Ackland, Biomechanical effects of fatigue on 10,000 meter running technique, *Research Quarterly for Exercise and Sport,* 52, 160–166, 1981.
17. Enoka, R.M., *Neuromechanics of Human Movement,* 3rd ed., Human Kinetics, Champaign, IL, 2001.
18. Fox, E.L., R.W. Bowers and M.L. Foss, *The Physiological Base or Exercise and Sport,* 5th ed., Brown and Benchmark, Madison, WI, 1993.
19. Fox, E.L., *Sport Physiology,* 2nd ed., Saunders College Publishing, New York, 1984.
20. Fox, E.L. and D.K. Mathews, *The Physiological Basis of Physical Education and Athletics,* 3rd ed., Saunders College Publishing, Philadelphia, 1981.
21. Gandevia, S.C., Spinal and supraspinal factors in human muscle fatigue, *Physiology Reviews,* 81, 1725–1789, 2001.
22. Hamill, J. and K.M. Knutzen, *Biomechanical Basis of Human Movement,* 2nd ed., Lippincott, Williams, and Wilkins, Philadelphia, 2003.
23. Hargraves, M., Exercise physiology and metabolism, in *Clinical Sports Nutrition,* 2nd ed., Burke. L. and V. Deakin, Eds., McGraw-Hill Book Company, New York, 2000.

24. Hargraves, M., Metabolic factors in fatigue, *Sports Science Exchange,* 18, 1–4, 2005.
25. Hoffman, J., *Physiological Aspects of Sport Training and Performance,* Human Kinetics, Champaign, IL, 2002.
26. Kirkendall, D.T., Fatigue from voluntary motor activity, in *Exercise and Sport Science,* Garrett, W.E. and D.T. Kirkendall, Eds., Lippincott, Williams, and Wilkins, Philadelphia, 2000.
27. Kraemer, W.J. and A.C. Fry, Strength testing: development and evaluation of methodology, in *Physiological Assessment of Human Fitness,* Maud, P.J. and C. Foster, Eds., Human Kinetics, Champaign, IL, 1995.
28. Kroll, W., Isometric strength fatigue patterns in female subjects, *Research Quarterly,* 42, 286–298, 1971.
29. Kroll, W. et al., Muscle fiber type composition and knee extension isometric strength fatigue patterns in power-and-endurance-trained males, *Research Quarterly for Exercise and Sport,* 51, 323–333, 1980.
30. Kroll, W., The 1981 C.H. McCloy Research Lecture: analysis of local muscular fatigue patterns, *Research Quarterly for Exercise and Sport,* 52, 523–539, 1981.
31. Laycoe, R.P. and R.G. Martiniuk, Learning and tension as factors in static strength gains produced by static and eccentric training, *Research Quarterly,* 42, 299–306, 1971.
32. Levangie, P.K. and C.C. Norkin, *Joint Structure and Function: A Comprehensive Analysis,* 4th ed., F.A. Davis Company, Philadelphia, 2005.
33. Magill, R.A., *Motor Learning: Concepts and Applications,* 7th ed., McGraw-Hill, New York, 2005.
34. McArdle, W.D., F.I. Katch, and V.L. Katch, Essentials of *Exercise Physiology,* 3rd ed., Lippincott, Williams, and Wilkins, Philadelphia, 2005.
35. Merton, P.A., Voluntary strength and fatigue, *Journal of Physiology,* 123, 553–564, 1954.
36. Nadel, E.R., Physiological adaptations to aerobic training, *American Scientist,* 73, 334–343, 1985.
37. Newsholme, E., Effects of exercise on aspects of carbohydrate, fat and amino acid metabolism, in *Exercise, Fitness and Health,* Bouchard, C., R. Shephard, and T. Stephens, Eds., Human Kinetics Publisher, Champaign, IL, 1990.
38. Newsholme, E., T. Leach, and B. Duester, *Keep on Running: The Science of Training and Performance,* John Wiley and Sons Limited, Chichester, England, 1993.
39. Nilsson, J., P. Tesch, and A. Thornstensson, Fatigue and E.M.G. of repeated fast voluntary contractions in man, *Acta Physiologica Scandinavica,* 101, 194–198, 1977.
40. Noakes, T., *Lore of Running,* 4th ed., Human Kinetics, Champaign, IL, 2002.
41. Nybo, L. and N.H. Secher, Cerebral perturbations provoked by prolonged exercise, *Progressive Neurobiology,* 2004.
42. Pack, M., D.J. Cotton and J. Biasotto, Effect of four fatigue levels on performance and learning of a novel balance skill, *Journal of Motor Behavior,* 6, 179–190, 1974.
43. Plowman, S.A. and D.L. Smith, *Exercise Physiology for Health, Fitness and Performance,* 2nd ed., Benjamin Cummings, San Francisco, 2003.
44. Powers, S.K. and E.T. Howley, *Exercise Physiology: Theory and Application to Fitness and Performance,* 5th ed., McGraw-Hill, New York, 2004.
45. Robergs, R.A. and S.J. Keteyian, Fundamentals of *Exercise Physiology for Fitness, Performance, and Health,* 2nd ed., McGraw-Hill, New York, 2003.
46. Rose, D.J., *A Multilevel Approach to the Study of Motor Control and Learning,* Allyn and Bacon, Boston, 1997.
47. Schmidt, R.A., *Motor Control and Learning: A Behavioral Emphasis,* 4th ed., Human Kinetics Publishers, Champaign, IL, 2005.

48. Segura, R. and J. Ventura, Effect of L-tryptophan supplementation on exercise performance, *International Journal of Sports Medicine,* 9, 301–305, 1988.
49. Sherman, W.M., Metabolism of sugars and physical performance, *American Journal of Clinical Nutrition,* 62, 228S–241S, 1995.
50. Singer, R.N., *Motor Learning and Human Performance,* 2nd ed., Macmillan Publishing Co., New York, 1975.
51. Snow, R.J. et al., Effect of carbohydrate ingestion on ammonia metabolism during exercise in humans, *Journal of Applied Physiology,* 88, 1576–1580, 2000.
52. Stone, M.H., Nutritional factors in performance and health, in *Essentials of Strength Training and Conditioning,* Baechle, T.R., Ed., Human Kinetics, Champaign, IL, 2000.
53. Stone, M.H. and M.S. Conley, Bioenergetics, in *Essentials of Strength Training and Conditioning,* Baechle, T.R., Ed., Human Kinetics, Champaign, IL, 2000.
54. Thorstensson, A. and J. Karlsson, Fatiguability and fiber composition of human skeletal muscle, *Acta Physiologica Scandinavica,* 98, 318–322, 1976.
55. Thorstensson, A., Muscle strength, fiber types, and enzyme activities in man, *Acta Physiologica Scandinavica Supplement,* 443, 1–45, 1976.
56. Todd, G. et al., Hyperthermia: a failure of the motor cortex and the muscle, *Journal of Physiology,* 563, 621–631, 2005.
57. Vander, A.J., J.H. Sherman, and D.S. Luciano, *Human Physiology: The Mechanisms of Body Function,* 5th ed., McGraw-Hill Publishing Company, New York, 1990.
58. Vandervalle, L. et al., Effect of branched-chain amino acid supplementation on exercise performance in glycogen depleted subjects, *Medicine and Science in Sport and Exercise,* 23, Supplement 116, 1991.
59. Vollestad, N.K. and O.M. Sijerstad, Biochemical correlates of fatigue, *European Journal of Applied Physiology,* 57, 336–347, 1988.
60. Welford, A.T., *Skill and Age,* Oxford University Press, London, 1951.
61. Welsh, R.S. et al., Carbohydrates and physical /mental performance during intermittent exercise in fatigue, *Medicine and Science in Sports and Exercise,* 34, 723–731, 2002.
62. Wilmore, J.H. and D.L. Costill, *Physiology of Sport and Exercise,* 3rd ed., Human Kinetics, Champaign, IL, 2004.
63. Wilson, G.J., Strength and power in sports, in *Applied Anatomy and Biomechanics in Sport,* Bloomfield, J., T.R. Ackland, and B.C. Elliott, Eds., Blackwell Scientific Publications, Melbourne, Australia, 1994.
64. Winnick, J.J. et al., Carbohydrate feedings during team sport exercise preserve physical and CNS function, *Medicine and Science in Sports and Exercise,* 37, 306–315, 2005.

Part Four

Nutrition and Heart Disease

8 Exercise and Nutrition

INTRODUCTION

Nutrition can be defined as the intake, transformation, and utilization of food substances. In relation to physical activity, nutrition provides the fundamental understandings to the physiological processes that occur during exercise relative to nutrient function. The basic nutrients include carbohydrates, fats, proteins, vitamins, minerals, and water. These nutrients are functionally used by the body for the following purposes:

1. energy metabolism
2. body tissue building and maintenance
3. regulation of bodily functions

CARBOHYDRATES

Carbohydrates are composed of carbon, hydrogen, and oxygen atoms in polysaccharide, disaccharide, and monosaccharide formations (Figure 8.1). Polysaccharides are the complex carbohydrates made up of starch, glycogen, and fiber. Disaccharides are simple carbohydrates such as sucrose, lactose, and maltose. Sucrose is a combination of glucose and fructose, lactose combines glucose and galactose, and maltose contains two molecules of glucose. Glucose, fructose, and galactose form the monosaccharides and are the end products of carbohydrate breakdown prior to their ultimate conversion to glucose in the liver. Complex carbohydrates are made up of these monosaccharide subunits in different atomic patterns, eventually breaking down to smaller and smaller simpler subunits. Glucose is the chief end product and serves as the major energy fuel for body metabolism and can be converted and stored as muscle and liver glycogen through the process of glycogenesis.

FATS

Fats are composed of carbon, hydrogen, and oxygen atoms and are classified as triglycerides, phospholipids, and sterols. Triglycerides form the predominant amount of fat in the body.[54] They break down to glycerol and three fatty acids through lipolytic degradation and undergo beta oxidation breakdown in mitochondrial acetyl coenzyme processes (Figure 8.2). Triglycerides are stored intramuscularly, in fat tissue, and in blood plasma. Phospholipids and sterols, namely cholesterol, constitute the remainder of the fat in the body. Glycogen, glycerol, and fatty acids provide

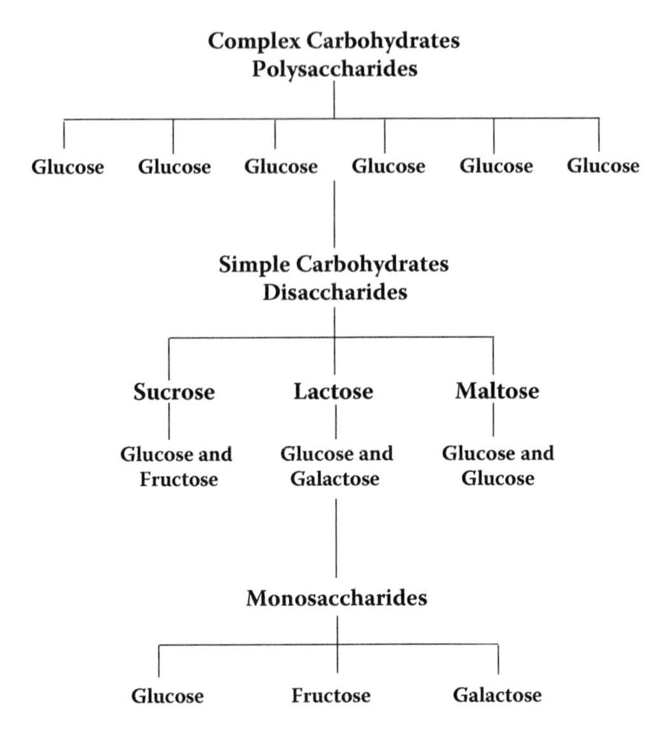

FIGURE 8.1 Carbohydrate structure.

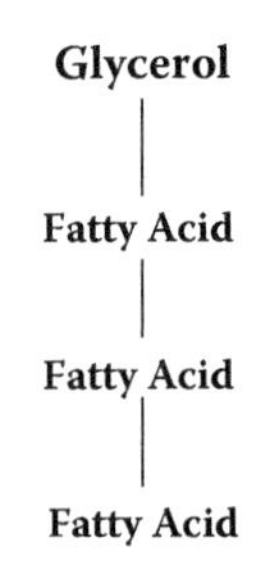

FIGURE 8.2 Triglyceride structure.

energy fuel for body metabolism. The energy from fat, however, is more concentrated and can be stored.

PROTEINS

Proteins are composed of carbon, oxygen, hydrogen, and nitrogen, and are constructed of linked chains of amino acids. Structurally, amino acids contain amino and acid groups attached to central carbon atoms with different side chains (Figure 8.3). The nitrogenous amino group is removed through deamination processes. The distinctive side chains identify amino acid differences. Amino acids form dipeptide

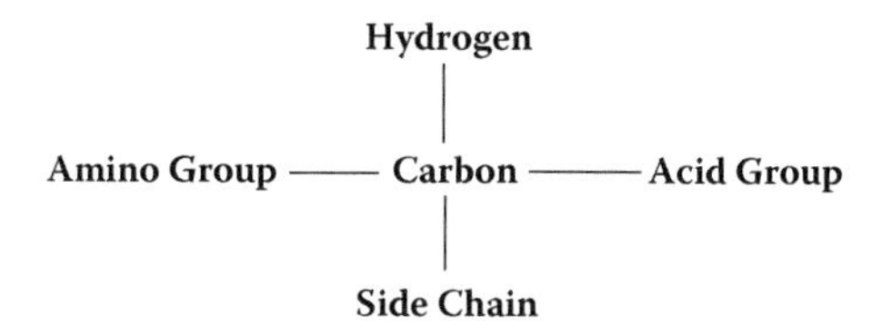

FIGURE 8.3 Protein structure.

Histidine
Isoleucine
Leucine
Lysine
Methionine
Phenylalanine
Threonine
Tryptophan
Valine

FIGURE 8.4 Essential amino acid figure.

(two), tripeptide (three), and polypeptide (many) linked chains through condensation processes. Oxygen and hydrogen are removed from one end of the acid group, and hydrogen is removed from the amino group, resulting in a bonding of the two amino acids. The removed hydrogen and oxygen also bond together to form water.

There are 20 amino acids, nine of which are termed to be essential (Figure 8.4). These amino acids cannot be synthesized in the body in sufficient quantities and must be included in the diet. The remaining amino acids can be formed in the body and are termed to be nonessential. Complete proteins contain the nine essential amino acids. Proteins can be used as direct and intermediate sources of energy. Amino acids can be oxidized through citric acid cycle and electron transport system processes and can also be converted to glucose and fat. The energy from protein is actively utilized in the body and not stored.

VITAMINS AND MINERALS

Vitamins are classified as organic compounds and act as biochemical catalysts in the transformation of food into energy. They contain carbon, hydrogen, oxygen, and in some instances nitrogen. When attached to proteins they serve as coenzymes and speed up the breakdown of fats, carbohydrates, and protein. Vitamins can be divided into water- and fat-soluble classifications (Figure 8.5). Water-soluble vitamins are absorbed through intestinal walls into the bloodstream. Fat-soluble vitamins, however, are emulsified much like fats before being absorbed through intestinal walls into the lymphatic system and then the bloodstream. While water-soluble vitamins are readily dissolved in the bloodstream, fat-soluble vitamins, like fat, must be carried by proteins in order to become soluble in the bloodstream. After utilization by cells, any excess intakes of water-soluble vitamins are excreted. In the case of

Fat Soluble Vitamins	Water Soluble Vitamins
	B-Complex Vitamins
Vitamin A	Thiamin (B1)
Vitamin D	Riboflavin (B2)
Vitamin E	Niacin (B3)
Vitamin K	Pyridoxine (B6)
	Folic Acid
	Pantothenic Acid
	Cobalamin (B12)
	Biotin
	Vitamin C

FIGURE 8.5 Fat- and water-soluble vitamins.

fat-soluble vitamins, excess intakes are stored in the body. Water-soluble vitamins include those of the B-complex and C, while the fat-soluble vitamins include A, D, E, and K. The B-complex vitamins can serve as coenzymes when attached to protein and can speed up the breakdown of food into energy.

Minerals are classified as inorganic substances and also act as regulatory agents in the body relative to nerve transmission, acid–base control, fluid balance, muscle contraction, and digestion.[5] Since they contain no carbon, minerals are inorganic and therefore do not break down in the body. Instead, they are composed of positive and negative ions and can combine with other ions, but still tend to retain their chemical nature. In reference to absorption, minerals are absorbed in the body much like water- and fat-soluble vitamins. Minerals can be divided into major and trace classifications (Figure 8.6). The major minerals include calcium, phosphorus, potassium, sulfur, sodium, chlorine, and magnesium. The trace minerals include iron, iodine, zinc, selenium, manganese, copper, molybdenum, cobalt, chromium, fluorine, silicon, vanadium, nickel, and tin.

Major Minerals	Trace Minerals
Calcium	Iron
Phosphorous	Iodine
Magnesium	Fluorine
Sulfur	Zinc
Sodium	Selenium
Potassium	Copper
Chloride	Cobalt
	Chromium
	Manganese
	Molybdenum
	Silicon
	Vanadium
	Nickel
	Tin

FIGURE 8.6 Major and trace minerals.

WATER

The water content in the body is mainly housed in intracellular (within cells) and extracellular (outside cells) compartments. Balance is maintained through osmotic pressure exchanges in and out of these two compartments. Water is absorbed through fluid intake, foods, and metabolic bodily processes and lost generally through urination, excretion, and perspiration. Body water contents are generally constant when intake equals output.

CARBOHYDRATE AND FAT UTILIZATION IN EXERCISE

The utilization of carbohydrates in exercise is generally determined by activity intensity and duration, training and muscle fiber type utilization, dietary composition, and glycogen concentration levels.[9,10,21,23,26,44] Glycogen and glucose utilization in exercise relative to intensity of effort is greatest when activity levels are strenuous.[4,54] Muscle glycogen is the primary energy contributor in the beginning stages of intense exercise, since it can be readily available for oxidation (Figure 8.7).[8] As exercise continues, glycogen is degraded to lactate, the lactate in turn is converted to glucose through glycogenolysis processes. At this point in time, muscle and liver glucose become the main sources of energy.[34] When carbohydrate depletion occurs, however,

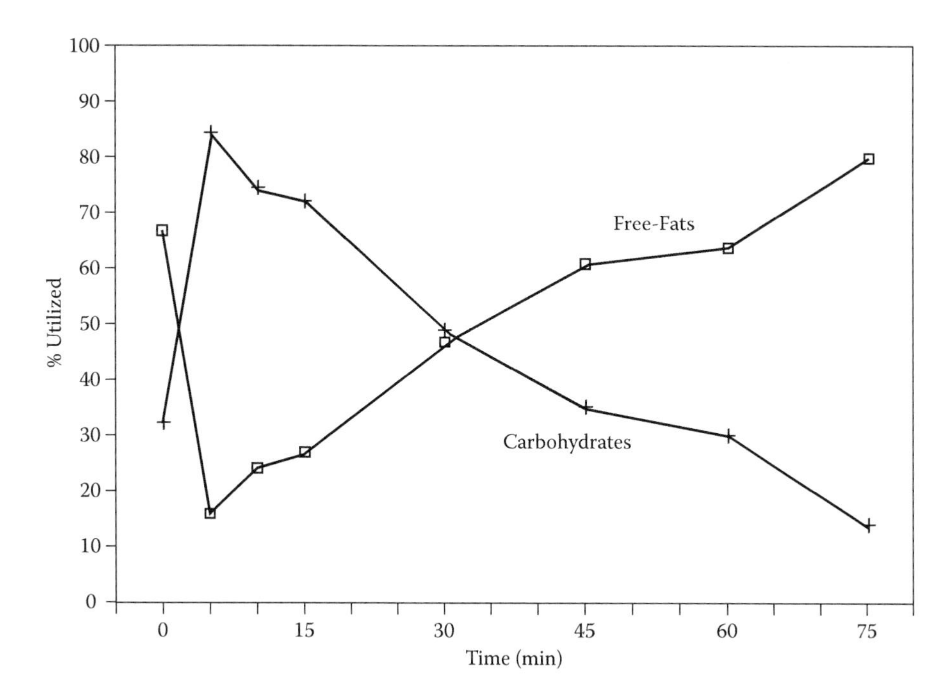

FIGURE 8.7 Utilization of carbohydrates and fats relative to performance time. (Adapted from Costill, D. *A Scientific Approach to Distance Running,* Tafnews Press, Los Altos, CA, 1979. With the permission of the publisher.)

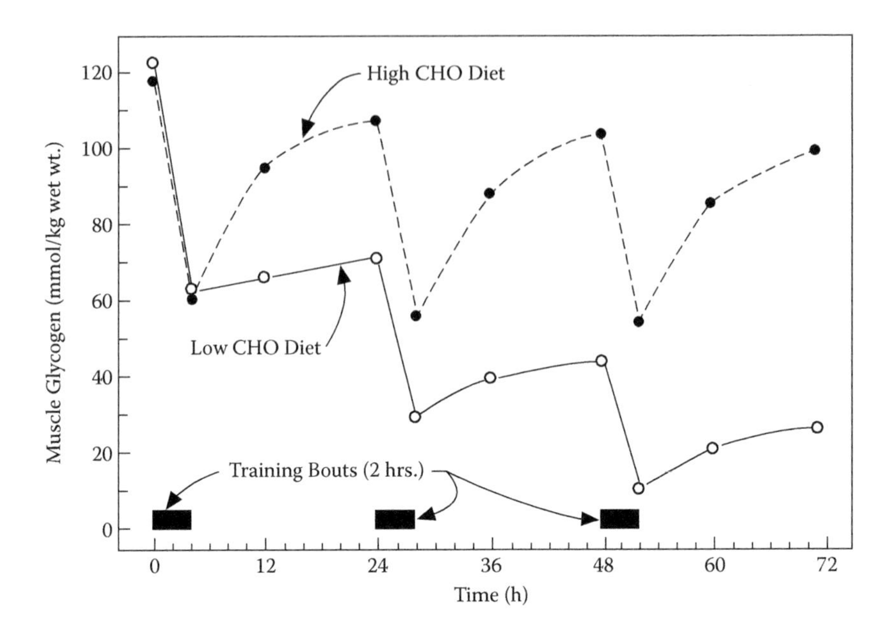

FIGURE 8.8 Muscle glycogen levels during heavy training: high (70%) and low (40%) carbohydrate diets. (From Costill, D.L. and J.M. Miller, *International Journal of Sports Medicine,* 1, 2–14, 1980. With the permission of Thieme Publishers, New York.)

fatigue eventually results, because limited amounts of carbohydrates are stored in the body. Further energy can be derived from gluconeogenesis processes in the formation of glucose from lactate, pyruvic acid, alanine, and glycerol.[45] The more strenuous the exercise level, the greater the carbohydrate depletion rate.[1,41] With an increase in exercise duration and a decrease in exercise intensity, fat becomes the major fuel source (Figure 8.8).[8] Intramuscular fat in the form of triglycerides is initially used, followed by the slow breakdown of blood fatty acids.[11,53] Later, as exercise duration continues, storage fatty acids are mobilized into the blood and are also used for energy purposes. Since more fat can be stored in the body, moderate levels of exercise intensity can be continued for greater lengths of time before fatigue sets in.[31] Fat may also play a more significant role in exercise intensity. Recent studies have shown that strenuous exercise results in a significant depletion of intramuscular fat.[40]

In reference to training state, the utilization of carbohydrate and fat differs.[3,5,35,39,40,49] With increased endurance training, the depletion rate of glycogen is slowed. There is a greater metabolic dependency upon fat as fuel. Slow- and fast-twitch muscle fibers proportionally increase their capacity to use fat, and deplete glycogen at slower rates.[26,28,37] Fast-twitch muscle fibers are primarily used during intensive exercise of short duration due to their greater glycolytic capacity.

Dietary composition relative to the intake of carbohydrates and fats also affects muscle and liver glycogen levels.[18,60] High carbohydrate diets, in comparison to high fat diets, result in greater exercise time to exhaustive fatigue due to greater levels of stored glycogen (Figure 8.8)[9,23,53]. High fat and high protein diets in this regard result in reduced glycogen content levels. In the past, carbohydrate loading was recommended to increase muscle and liver glycogen levels. The classic description of carbohydrate loading included the depletion of glycogen stores through exhaustive exercise, the intake of fats and protein for three days, and the consumption of large amounts of carbohydrates for the three days preceding competition.[37,60] The results of this process would be the supersaturation of muscle and liver glycogen. This practice, however, can be potentially dangerous and may result in cardiac abnormalities, muscle cell damage, an increase in triglyceride levels, feelings of heaviness and stiffness, and hypoglycemia.[41]

Recent evidence, however, has demonstrated that glycogen storage can be increased and maintained comparatively through modified dietary intake practices.[38,43,48,51,52] In this regard, the Food and Nutrition Board of the Institute of Medicine proposed new macronutrient range intakes of 45–65% for carbohydrate, 20–35% for fat, and 10–35% for protein based on energy needs relative to age, gender, body size, and activity level.[21,44] The use of these dietary intake macronutrient ranges would modify the carbohydrate loading practices of the past. The moderate-intensity and high-intensity activity ranges proposed for carbohydrates were 5–7 and 7–12 grams per kilogram of body weight, respectively. Protein intake levels ranged from 1.2 to 1.7 grams per kilogram of body weight, and fat consumption requirements ranged from 20 to 35% relative to the intake of low saturated fat and adequate amounts of the essential fatty acids.

Studies on athletic training and performance have also noted the continuous need for carbohydrate intake before, during, and after endurance or intensive activities in order to maintain high levels of glycogen in the body.[9,23,30,36,53] In reference to preexercise practices, the recently developed glycemic index may be used as a guide. (Figure 8.9).[12,46,50,55,56,59] The glycemic index ranks the bodily absorption rate of foods that produce a high, moderate, or low rise in blood sugar. High glycemic foods generally include sugars, syrups, and jellies, while moderate and low glycemic foods include vegetables, legumes, dairy products, and fruit. However, since the glycemic index applies to single foods and not to mixed foods, any calculation can be erroneous. In addition, some carbohydrates may be indexed as low and some as moderate or high. The glycemic load corrects these differences through the use of the index percentage multiplied by the actual amount of carbohydrates in grams consumed.[35,55] Glycemic loads are ranked as low (ten or less), moderate (eleven to nineteen), and high (twenty or more).[55] High glycemic load foods break down quickly, and when taken one hour before a long endurance run, can contribute to hyperglycemic/hypoglycemic reactions. Blood glucose rises quickly and can create a hyperglycemic effect. However, after insulin is released from the pancreas, blood glucose is carried to the body cells for use and, in the process, can create a drop in blood sugar levels, resulting in a hypoglycemic reaction. This reaction may not occur if low to moderate glycemic load foods are consumed, since the hyperglycemic/hypoglycemic effects would be slowed or minimized.[53,55,60] Fructose intake before exercise may also elicit minimal hypoglycemic reactions, since it is absorbed more slowly before converting to glucose.[12] High fructose concentration intake, however, should not be encouraged, because of the possibility of gastrointestinal discomfort.[4] Generally, complex carbohydrates foods are digested more slowly in the body and therefore do not elicit quick

High Glycemic Index (>85)	Medium Glycemic Index (60–85)	Low Glycemic Index (<60)
Glucose	All-Bran Cereal	Fructose
Sucrose	Banana	Apple
Maple syrup	Grapes	Applesauce
Corn syrup	Oatmeal	Cherries
Honey	Orange juice	Kidney beans
Bagel	Pasta	Navy beans
Candy	Rice	Chick-peas
Corn flakes	Whole-grain rye bread	Lentils
Carrots	Yams	Dates
Crackers	Corn	Figs
Molasses	Baked beans	Peaches
Potatoes	Potato chips	Plums
Raisins		Ice cream
Bread, white and whole wheat		Milk
Soda, with sugar		Yogurt
Sports drinks with sugar		Tomato soup
Exceed		
Gatorade		
Sports drinks with polymers		
Gatorlode		
Exceed High Carbohydrate		

FIGURE 8.9 Glycemic index of common foods. (From Williams, M.H., *Nutrition for Fitness and Sport,* 4th ed., Brown and Benchmark, Madison, WI, 1995. Reproduced with the permission of McGraw-Hill Companies.)

hypoglycemic reactions. During exercise, carbohydrate and carbohydrate fluid solutions should be consumed early for either long endurance or intensive activities so as to promote absorption and maintain glycogen and glucose levels.[23,53] In the postexercise period, carbohydrate and protein intake should begin early in order to promote glycogen storage and protein synthesis.[23,51]

PROTEIN AND PERFORMANCE

With the breakdown of protein to amino acids, pools of amino acids are formed in tissue and blood. In these pools, amino acids are synthesized and degraded when complete protein needs are met and used for structural and bodily purposes. Other amino acids not utilized in this manner can be oxidized and used as fuel for energy or converted to glucose and fatty acids (glycogenic and ketogenic amino acids) and also used as sources of energy. The branched-chain amino acids leucine, isoleucine, and valine are oxidized in muscle tissue.[1,4]

Recent research has indicated that protein utilization may be metabolically regulated by carbohydrate depletion and by the rate of amino acid degradation during exercise (Figure 8.10). Evans and Hughes[18] and Evans et al.[20] found that protein synthesis decreases and protein degradation increases during exercise. This

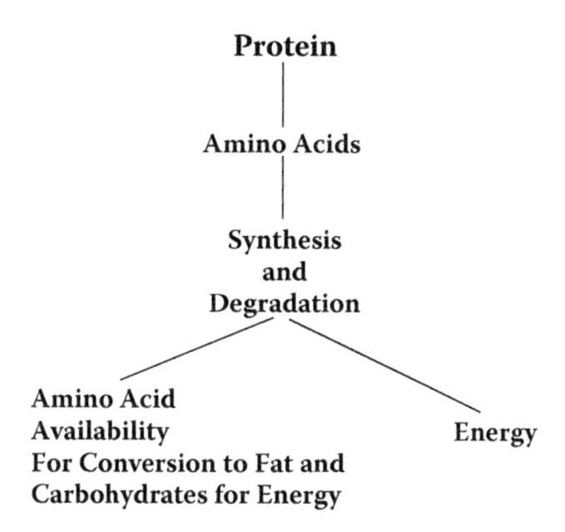

FIGURE 8.10 Generalized summary of protein synthesis and degradation during exercise.

process is continuous in nature and regulated by exercise intensity and amino acid availability.[4,34] An increase in amino acid availability could therefore result in an increase in glucose and fatty acid oxidation rates, an increase in the amount of amino acid conversion to glucose, and an increase in amino acid breakdown for muscle tissue utilization.[4,13,14,33,34,39]

While the daily recommended allowance for protein has been set at 0.8 g/kg body weight, the intake of additional protein has become a common practice among athletes who train on an intensive level for conditioning purposes. Lemon,[32–34] in his studies on protein and exercise, advocated that strength, speed, and endurance male and female athletes should take in 1.6 to 1.8 and 1.2 to 1.4 grams of protein per kilogram of body weight, respectively. These intake ranges would be representative of a 10 to 15% dietary protein allowance. Ellsworth et al.[17] found protein utilization to range from 13.2 to 14.2% for elite male and 12.7 to 14.3% for elite female Nordic skiers.

Excessive protein intake levels, however, can be toxic because urea and ammonia are also by-products of protein metabolism.[24] These waste by-products circulate in the body until they are filtered through the kidneys and excreted. Recent research has also noted that excessive protein intakes could result in ketosis, dehydration, calcium loss, gout, and kidney stress.[6,25,37]

VITAMIN AND MINERAL UTILIZATION IN EXERCISE

The supplemental utilization of vitamins and minerals to improve performance has been an area of controversy. Vitamins and minerals in general regulate metabolic processes and are involved in the transformation of food into energy. Adequate dietary intake of both vitamins and minerals is essential to the physiologic function of the body during exercise. Deficiencies in this regard have been related to decreased physical performance.[30,57] These deficiencies, however, can be normalized through additional dietary intake of foods containing the designated vitamins and minerals.[2,19] In reference to the supplemental utilization of vitamins and minerals, Costill[9] reported that such practices aimed at the improvement of performance were not justifiable. Research in this area of study tends to corroborate this point of view.[45,51,60] For example, vitamins B, C, and E have been studied in this regard because they play a role in fat and carbohydrate metabolism, oxidative energy availability, and endurance performance.[1,4] In reference to B-complex supplementation, exercise studies on thiamin, riboflavin, and niacin, which are primarily associated with energy metabolism, have generally not shown an ability to enhance metabolic capacity.[37,46,52,58,60] Similarly, studies on the effect of vitamin C supplementation on oxygen availability to muscle tissues during exercise have also not shown an ability to improve oxidative capacity.[37,57,60] In regard to E, a fat-soluble vitamin, and increased endurance performance capacity, studies have not demonstrated significant evidence in this regard.[9,37] It should be noted that since vitamin E is a fat-soluble vitamin and is stored in the body, care must be taken with supplemental ingestion, because toxicity may result. Recent studies have also shown that large dosages of vitamin C, a water-soluble vitamin, can result in nausea, abdominal cramps, and diarrhea.[37]

There is also little support for the supplementation of minerals relative to exercise losses.[4,7,43] Reported losses of calcium, magnesium, sodium, potassium, and chloride during performance generally were replaceable through dietary means. In reference to iron deficiency, the evidence is somewhat mixed. Iron deficiency can be related to a condition known as sports anemia. As a result, significant aerobic decreases in physical performance may occur.[37,57,60] Iron supplements may be of value under these circumstances.[37] However, iron supplements may not provide the answer, since endurance studies show this relationship may be more a matter of physiological response to training.[54] Low levels of hematocrit in athletes may, in essence, belie a high total blood volume and higher hemoglobin levels.[29,41] Iron deficiency may also be a result of inadequate iron intake.[27] Additional dietary intake of iron may be warranted in this case, since iron loss in exercise through perspiration occurs during endurance training.[16] Iron losses under these circumstances, however, may not be significant. Dressendorfer et al.,[15] in their study on plasma mineral levels in marathoners, did not find iron reduction in runners to be persistent after a 312-mile, 20-day road race.

WATER AND EXERCISE

The utilization of water increases during periods of physical activity. Water loss occurs mainly through the loss of heat through sweat evaporation, urine and feces, and in air exhalation.[43] Even though water production is increased during exercise through oxidative metabolic processes, water loss begins to exceed this increase when intensity levels rise. Without fluid replacement, dehydration can occur, and performance can be affected. Water hydration and replacement levels have been generally set at 150 to 350 ml every 15–20 minutes during exercise.[6,42] Dehydration can occur, and water replacement is recommended.

In reference to fluids other than water, electrolyte replacement and carbohydrate loading drink solutions are generally used to provide energy and to maintain the necessary fluid hydrated balance for exercise and activity sessions.[10] Electrolytic replacement drinks (sodium, potassium, and chloride) are used primarily to maintain levels of these nutrients due to perspiration losses.[60] Solutions of 6 to 8% are used, and ingestion is determined by the intensity and duration of exercise.[22,47,59] Carbohydrate loading drinks (sucrose, glucose, fructose, and maltodextrin) are used primarily to supplement the depletion of muscle glycogen levels and to promote glycogen synthesis in an effort to delay the onset of fatigue.[8,22] Fluid replacement and carbohydrate loading drink solutions are to be ingested before, during, and after short, medium, and long intensive and endurance exercise periods of work. Dehydration, gastric emptying, and intestinal absorption are the significant fluid determinants. According to Gisolfi and Duchman,[22] intake of these fluids should range from 300 to 500 ml, 15 min before an activity, 800 to 1600 ml per hour for an activity lasting 1 to 3 hours, and 500 to 1000 ml per hour for an activity lasting beyond 3 hours.

SUMMARY

In summary, the conclusions that can be drawn from these studies indicated that:

1. Carbohydrates, fats, proteins, vitamins, and minerals are used by the body for the purposes of energy metabolism, body tissue building and maintenance, and body function regulation.
2. In reference to carbohydrates, glucose serves as the major energy fuel for body metabolism in the forms of blood glucose and muscle and liver glycogen.
3. Fats, in the form of glycerol and fatty acids, provide energy fuel for body metabolism. The energy fuel from fat, however, is more concentrated and can be stored.
4. Proteins are utilized as an intermediate source of energy. Amino acids can be converted to glucose and fat and/or oxidized through citric acid cycle and electron transport system processes.
5. Vitamins and minerals are classified as organic and inorganic compounds, respectively, and act as biochemical catalysts in the transformation of food into energy.
6. The water content in the body is mainly housed in intracellular and extracellular compartments. Balance is maintained through osmotic pressure exchanges in and out of these two compartments.
7. The utilization of carbohydrates and fat in exercise is generally determined by activity (intensity and duration), by level of training and muscle fiber utilization, and by dietary composition and glycogen concentration levels.
8. The use of protein as an energy source is limited and related to the availability of carbohydrates and fats.
9. The supplemental utilization of vitamins and minerals for the improvement of performance has not been justified.
10. Water utilization increases during periods of exercise. Water loss occurs mainly through the loss of heat through sweat evaporation.
11. Electrolyte replacement and carbohydrate loading drink solutions are generally used to provide energy and to maintain the necessary fluid hydrated balance for exercise and activity sessions.

GLOSSARY

Amino acids The basic structure of proteins that contain amino and acid groups attached to central carbon atoms with different side chains

Beta oxidation Fatty acid oxidation through mitochondrial acetyl coenzyme energy processes

Carbohydrate loading drinks Solutions containing sucrose, fructose, glucose, and maltodextrin used to replace these nutrients during exercise

Carbohydrates Compounds that contain carbon, hydrogen, and oxygen atoms in polysaccharide, disaccharide, and monosaccharide formations

Cholesterol A sterol, an essential metabolite, and a fat-like substance

Chylomicrons Lipoproteins that are large in size, light in weight, and contain triglycerides

Deamination The process of nitrogenous amino group removal from protein

Diglycerides Fat compounds that contain glycerol and two fatty acids

Disaccharides Simple carbohydrates such as sucrose, lactose, and maltose

Electrolyte replacement Solutions containing sodium, potassium, and chloride to replace depletion of these nutrients during exercise

Fats Compounds that contain carbon, hydrogen, and oxygen and are classified as triglycerides, phospholipids, and cholesterol.

Glucose The basic carbohydrate unit that serves as a major energy fuel

Glycemic index A classification index that ranks the bodily absorption rate of foods that produce a high, moderate, or low rise in blood sugar

Glycemic load The glycemic index percentage multiplied by the actual amount of carbohydrate in grams consumed

Glycogen The stored form of glucose in muscle and liver tissue

Glycogenesis The process of glycogen formation from glucose

Glycogenolysis The process of glucose formation from glycogen

Glyconeogenesis The process of glucose formation through the conversion of lactate, pyruvic acid, alanine, and glycerol

High-density lipoproteins Lipoproteins that are small in size, dense in weight, and are the main carriers of cholesterol from body tissues

Hyperglycemic reactions The rise in blood sugar following the intake of simple carbohydrates

Hypoglycemic reactions The drop in blood sugar following the release of insulin, which drives the sugar to the body cells

Lipoproteins Water soluble protein and phospholipid carriers of triglycerides and cholesterol through the bloodstream

Low-density lipoproteins Lipoproteins that contain mostly cholesterol and are the prime carriers of this sterol to body tissues

Minerals Inorganic substances that act as regulatory agents in the body

Monoglycerides Fat compounds that contain glycerol and one fatty acid

Monosaccharides Simple carbohydrates such as glucose, fructose, and galactose

Monounsaturated fats Fats that contain one double bond per molecule

Phospholipids Fat compounds that contain two fatty acids and one phosphoric acid with a nitrogenous base

Polysaccharides Complex carbohydrates that include starches, sugars, and fiber

Polyunsaturated fats Fats that have more than one double bond per molecule

Proteins Compounds that contain carbon, hydrogen, and oxygen and are constructed of linked chains of amino acids

Saturated fats Fats that carry all of the hydrogen possible relative to carbon atom attachment

Triglycerides Fat compounds that contain glycerol and three fatty acids

Very low-density lipoproteins Lipoproteins that are partially degraded chylomicrons and contain mostly triglycerides

Vitamins Organic compounds that act as biochemical catalysts in the transformation of food into energy

REFERENCES

1. Adams, A.K. and T.M. Best, The role of antioxidants in exercise and disease prevention, *The Physician and Sports Medicine,* 30, May, 2002.
2. Armstrong, L.E. and C.M. Maresh, Vitamin and mineral supplements as nutritional aids to exercise performance and health, *Nutrition Reviews,* 54, S149–S158, 1996.
3. Bouchard, C., R.J. Shephard, and T. Stephens, Editors, *Physical Activity, Fitness, and Health: Consensus Statement,* Human Kinetics Publishers, Champaign, IL, 1993.
4. Brouns, F. and C. Cargill, *Essentials of Sports Nutrition,* 2nd ed., John Wiley and Sons, New York, 2002.
5. Brown, J.E., *Nutrition Now,* 2nd ed., Wadsworth Publishing Company, Belmont, CA, 1999.
6. Casa, D.J. et al., National Athletic Trainers' Association Position Statement, Fluid replacement for athletes, *Journal of Athletic Training,* 35, 212–224, 2000.
7. Coggan, A. and E.F. Coyle, Carbohydrate ingestion during prolonged exercise: effects on metabolism and performance, in *Exercise and Sports Sciences Reviews,* Holloszy, J.O., Ed., Williams and Wilkins, Baltimore, 1991.
8. Costill, D.L., *A Scientific Approach to Distance Running,* Track and Field News, Los Altos, CA, 1979.
9. Costill, D.L. and J.M. Miller, Nutrition for endurance sport: carbohydrates and fluid balance, *International Journal of Sport Medicine,* 1, 2–14, 1980; Carbohydrate for athletic training and performance, *Contemporary Nutrition,* 15, 1–2, 1990.
10. Coyle, E.F., Fluid and fuel intake during exercise, *Journal of Sports Science,* 22, 39–55, 2004.
11. Coyle, E.F., Fat metabolism during exercise, *Sports Science Exchange,* 8, 1–5, 1995.
12. Coyle, E.F. and E. Coyle, Carbohydrates that speed recovery from training, *The Physician and Sports Medicine,* 21, 111–123, February, 1993.
13. DiPasquale, M., *Amino Acids and Proteins for the Athlete: The Anabolic Edge,* CRC Press, Boca Raton, FL, 1997.
14. Dohm, G.L., Protein nutrition for the athlete, *Clinics in Sports Medicine,* 3, 595–604, 1984.
15. Dressendorfer, R.C. et al., Plasma mineral levels in marathon runners during a 20-day road race, *The Physician and Sports Medicine,* 10, 113–118, 1982.
16. Ehn, L., B. Carlmark, and S. Hoglund, Iron status in athletes involved in intense physical activity, *Medicine,* 10, 113–118, 1982.

17. Ellsworth, N.M., B.F. Hewitt, and W.L. Haskell, Nutrient intake of elite male and female nordic skiers, *The Physician and Sports Medicine,* 13, 78–92, 1995.
18. Evans, W.J. and V.A. Hughes, Dietary carbohydrates and endurance exercise, *The American Journal of Clinical Nutrition,* 41, 1146–1154, May, 1985.
19. Evans, W. and I.H. Rosenburg with J. Thompson, *Biomarkers: The 10 Determinants of Aging You Can Control,* Simon and Schuster, New York, 1995.
20. Evans, W.J. et al., Protein metabolism and endurance exercise, *The Physician and Sports Medicine,* 11, 63–72, 1983.
21. Food and Nutrition Board, Institute of Medicine, Dietary reference intakes, Energy, carbohydrates, fiber, fat, fatty acids, cholesterol, proteins, and amino acids, National Academy Press, Washington, DC, 2002.
22. Gisolfi, C.V. and S.M. Duchman, Guidelines for optimal replacement beverages for different athletic events, *Medicine and Science in Sports and Exercise,* 24, 679–687, 1992.
23. Hargraves, M., Carbohydrate metabolism and exercise, in *Exercise and Sport Science,* Garrett, W.F. Jr. and D.T. Kirkendall, Eds., Lippincott, Williams, and Wilkins, Philadelphia, 2000.
24. Heck, K., Nutrition, diet, and weight control for athletes, *Journal of Physical Education and Recreation,* 51, 43–45, June, 1980.
25. Heyward, V.H., *Advanced Fitness Assessment and Exercise Prescription,* 2nd ed., Human Kinetics Books, Champaign, IL, 1991.
26. Hickson, R.C., *Carbohydrate Metabolism in Exercise,* Report of the Ross Symposium on Nutrient Utilization During Exercise, Tarpon Springs, FL, November, 1982.
27. Hoeger, W.W.K. and S.A. Hoeger, *Principles and Labs for Fitness and Wellness,* 6th ed., Wadsworth/ Thomson Learning, Belmont, CA, 2001.
28. Holloszy, J.O., Muscle metabolism during exercise, *Archives of Physical Medicine and Rehabilitation,* 63, 231–233, May, 1982.
29. Katch, F.I. and W.D. McArdle, *Introduction to Nutrition, Exercise, and Health,* 4rth ed., Lea and Febiger, Malvern, PA, 1993.
30. Lamb, D.R., Basic principles for improving sports performance, *Sports Science Exchange,* 8, 1–5, 1995.
31. Lambert, E.V. et al., Nutritional strategies for promoting fat utilization and delaying the onset of fatigue during prolonged exercise, *Journal of Sport Science,* 15, 315–324, 1997.
32. Lemon, P.W.R., Is Increased dietary protein necessary or beneficial for individuals with a physically active lifestyle? *Nutrition Reviews,* 54, S169–S175, 1996.
33. Lemon, P.W.R., Beyond the Zone: protein needs of active individuals, *Journal of the American College of Nutrition,* 19, 513S–521S, 2000.
34. Lemon, P.W.R., Protein metabolism during exercise, in *Exercise and Sport Science,* Garrett, W.F. Jr., and D.T. Kirkendall, Eds., Lippincott, Williams, and Wilkins, Philadelphia, 2000.
35. Ludwig, D.S., The glycemic index: physiological mechanisms relating to obesity, diabetes, and cardiovascular disease, *Journal of the American Medical Association,* 287, 2414–2423, May 8, 2003.
36. Macdonald, I., Sugars for success? *British Journal of Sports Medicine,* 24, 93–94, June, 1990.
37. Mahan, L.K. and M. Arlin, Nutrition for athletic training and performance, in *Krause's Food, Nutrition, and Diet Therapy,* Mahan, L.K. and M. Arlin, Eds., W.B. Saunders Company, Philadelphia, 1992.

38. Manore, M.M., Nutrition and physical activity: fueling the active individual, *Research Digest*, President's Council on Physical Fitness and Sports, Series 5, No, 1, 1–8, March, 2004.
39. McArdle, W.D., F.I. Katch and V.L. Katch, *Exercise Physiology: Energy, Nutrition, and Human Performance,* 6th ed., Lippincott, Williams, and Wilkins, Philadelphia, 2006.
40. Muoio, D.M. et al., Effect of dietary fat on metabolic adjustments to maximal VO_2 and endurance in runners, *Medicine and Science in Sports and Exercise,* 26, 81–88, 1994.
41. Newsholme, E., T. Leech and G. Duester, *Keep On Running: The Science of Training and Performance,* John Wiley and Sons Ltd., West Sussex, England, 1994.
42. Nieman, D.C., *Fitness and Sports Medicine: A Health-Related Approach,* 3rd ed., Bull Publishing Company, Palo Alto, CA, 1995.
43. Nutrition: Got water? *Harvard Health Letter,* 28, 1–8, August, 2001.
44. Position of the American Dietetic Association and the Canadian Dietetic Association: nutrition for physical fitness and athletic performance for adults, *Journal of the American Dietetic Association,* 93, 691–695, 1993.
45. Powers, S.K. and E.T. Howley, *Exercise Physiology: Theory and Application to Fitness and Performance,* 5th ed., McGraw-Hill, New York, 2004.
46. Rankin, J.W., Glycemic index and exercise metabolism, *Sports Science Exchange,* 10, 1–8, 1997.
47. Rockwell, M., Fluid dynamics, *Training and Conditioning,* 16, May–June, 2006.
48. Shirreffs, S.M., L.E. Armstrong, and S.N. Cheuvront, Fluid and electrolyte needs for preparation and recovery from training and competition, *Journal of Sports Science,* 22, 57–63, 2004.
49. Simopoulos, A.P., Nutrition and fitness: A conference report, *Nutrition Today,* 29, 24–29, November/December, 1992.
50. Stone, M.H. Nutritional factors in performance and health, in *Essentials of Strength Training and Conditioning,* Baechle, T.R., Ed., Human Kinetics, Champaign, IL, 1994.
51. Suzuki, M., Glycemic carbohydrates consumed with amino acids or protein right after exercise enhance muscle formation, *Nutrition Reviews,* 61, S88-S94, May, 2003.
52. Virk, R.S. et al., Effect of vitamin B-6 supplementation on fuels, catecholamines, and amino acids during exercise in men, *Medicine and Science in Sports and Exercise,* 31, 400–407, 1999.
53. Volek, J.S., Enhancing exercise performance: nutritional implications, in *Exercise and Sport Science,* Garrett, W.F. Jr., and D.T. Kirkendall, Eds., Lippincott, Williams, and Wilkins, Philadelphia, 2000.
54. Whitney, E.N. and S.R. Rolfes, *Understanding Nutrition,* 10th ed., West Wadsworth, Belmont, CA, 2005.
55. Whyte, J.J., The glycemic index: How useful is it? *Consultant,* 45, 558–559 April 15, 2005.
56. Williams, M.H., *Nutritional Aspects of Human Physical and Athletic Performance,* 2nd ed., Charles C. Thomas, Springfield, IL, 1985.
57. Williams, M.H., Vitamin and mineral supplements to athletes: Do they help? Symposium on Nutritional Aspects of Exercise, *Clinics in Sports Medicine,* 3, 623–637, July, 1984.
58. Williams, M.H., Vitamin, iron, and calcium supplementation: effect on human physical performance, nutrition and athletic performance, *Proceedings of the Conference on Nutritional Determinants in Athletic Performance,* San Francisco, CA, September 24–25, 1981.

59. Williams, M.H., *Nutrition for Health, Fitness and Sport,* 6th ed., McGraw-Hill, New York, 2002.
60. Wilmore, J.H. and D.L. Costill, *Physiology of Sport and Exercise,* 3rd ed., Human Kinetics, Champaign, IL, 2004.

9 Nutrition and Heart Disease

INTRODUCTION

The relationship of total cholesterol to the development of atherosclerosis and heart disease has been substantially studied. Epidemiological and cross-cultural investigations of this nature have generally demonstrated a positive causal relationship between cholesterol and the prevalence of heart disease.[13,14,35,52,81,83,100] Evidence in this regard has centered on a lipid hypothesis that relates:[36,63,68,83]

1. Saturated fat intake and cholesterol
2. Saturated fat intake and serum lipid levels
3. Serum lipid levels, cholesterol, and heart disease
4. Lowered cholesterol intake and heart disease risk reduction

LIPIDS AND LIPOPROTEINS

The major lipid components in blood are triglycerides, phospholipids, and cholesterol. Triglycerides, the predominant fat content in the body, are compound structures of glycerol and three fatty acids[99] (Figure 9.1). Glycerol attached to one or two fatty acids is referred to, respectively, as monoglycerides and diglycerides. Both of these fats act as emulsifiers in the body. Fatty acids can be classified according to carbon atom number and hydrogen saturation (Figure 9.2). In reference to number, fatty acids with less than 8 carbon atoms are termed to be short chained, between 8 and 16 are medium chained, and over 16 are long chained. Carbon atoms also differ in regard to hydrogen molecule saturation. Saturated fatty acids have all the hydrogen atoms the carbon atoms can hold, while monounsaturated and polyunsaturated fatty acids substitute double bonds between carbon atoms for two or more hydrogen atoms, respectively. Missing hydrogen bonds on the same side of the double bond between carbon atoms are referred to as cis, while missing bonds on both sides are termed trans fatty acids.

Phospholipids and cholesterol form the remainder of the fat in the body. Phospholipids are made up of glycerol, two fatty acids, and one phosphoric acid with a nitrogenous base (Figure 9.3). They are termed fat emulsifiers because of their insoluble/soluble integrative reaction to water. Cholesterol, a sterol, is an essential metabolite and a complex fat (Figure 9.4). Functionally, cholesterol is a component of cell membranes, bile acids, steroid hormones, and vitamin D.[80] The body obtains

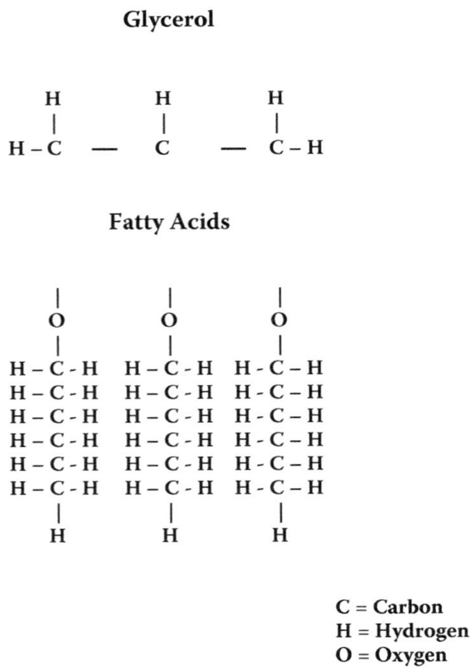

Glycerol

```
 H         H         H
 |         |         |
H-C   —    C    —    C-H
```

Fatty Acids

```
  |       |       |
  O       O       O
  |       |       |
H-C-H   H-C-H   H-C-H
H-C-H   H-C-H   H-C-H
H-C-H   H-C-H   H-C-H
H-C-H   H-C-H   H-C-H
H-C-H   H-C-H   H-C-H
H-C-H   H-C-H   H-C-H
  |       |       |
  H       H       H
```

C = Carbon
H = Hydrogen
O = Oxygen

FIGURE 9.1 Triglyceride structure.

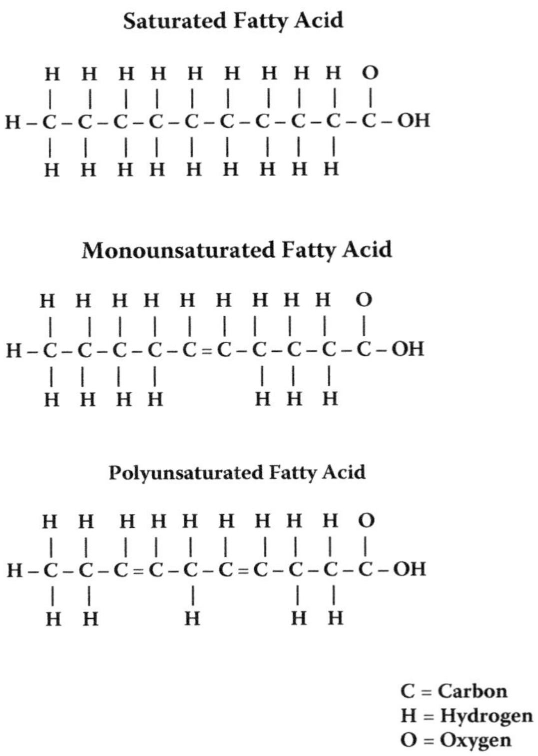

Saturated Fatty Acid

```
  H H H H H H H H H O
  | | | | | | | | | |
H-C-C-C-C-C-C-C-C-C-C-OH
  | | | | | | | | |
  H H H H H H H H H
```

Monounsaturated Fatty Acid

```
  H H H H H H H H H O
  | | | | | | | | | |
H-C-C-C-C-C=C-C-C-C-C-OH
  | | | |     | | |
  H H H H     H H H
```

Polyunsaturated Fatty Acid

```
  H H H H H H H H H O
  | | | | | | | | | |
H-C-C-C=C-C-C=C-C-C-C-OH
  | |     |     | |
  H H     H     H H
```

C = Carbon
H = Hydrogen
O = Oxygen

FIGURE 9.2 Saturated, monounsaturated, and polyunsaturated acid structures.

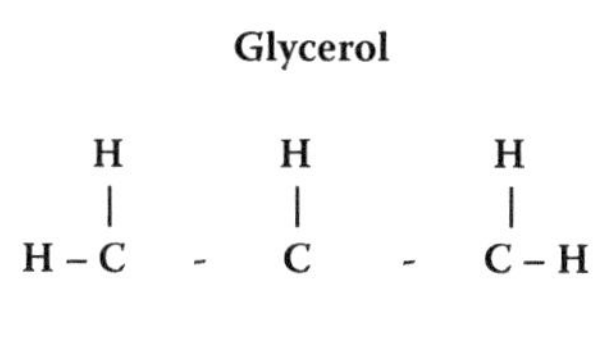

Fatty Acids

H – O – H H – O – H **Phosphoric Acid with a Nitrogenous Base**
H – C – H H – C – H
H – C – H H – C – H
H – C – H H – C – H
H – C – H H – C – H
H – C – H H – C – H
H – C – H H – C – H
H – C – H H – C – H
H H

C = Carbon
H = Hydrogen
O = Oxygen

FIGURE 9.3 Phospholipid structure.

CH_3 CH_3 CH_3 CH_3 CH_3 HO

FIGURE 9.4 Cholesterol.

cholesterol through endogenous production and exogenous intake. The liver produces approximately 85%, while dietary intake accounts for the remaining 15%.[100] Total cholesterol levels are influenced by dietary intake, liver synthesis, absorption percentage, transport breakdown, and excretion.[80]

The transportation of these major blood lipids is dependent upon plasma lipoproteins, since they are insoluble in watery solutions. Lipoproteins or fat-carrying proteins form water-soluble coverings around these lipids in order to carry them to the lymph nodes and blood (Figure 9.5).[97,98] There are basically four major types of lipoproteins which are classified according to increasing density, protein and phospholipid concentrations, and decreasing triglyceride makeup.[37,99] These four major classes are:

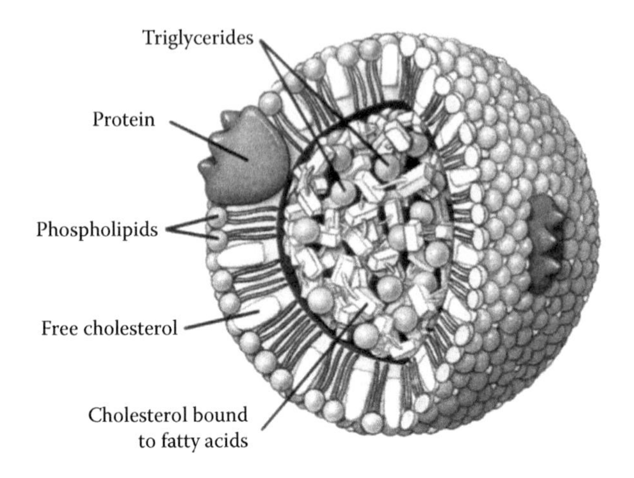

FIGURE 9.5 Lipoprotein structure (LDL). (From Wardlaw, G. *Contemporary Nutrition,* 3rd ed., Brown and Benchmark, Madison, WI, 1997. Reproduced with the permission of the McGraw-Hill Companies.)

1. Chylomicrons — These lipoproteins are large in size, light in weight, and contain mostly triglycerides.
2. Very low-density lipoproteins (VLDL) — These fat-carrying proteins are partially degraded chylomicrons and contain mostly triglycerides.
3. Low-density lipoproteins (LDL) — These lipoproteins contain mostly cholesterol and are the prime carriers of this sterol to body tissues.
4. High-density lipoproteins (HDL) — These fat carrying proteins are small in size and dense in weight. They are produced separately in the liver and are the main carriers of cholesterol from the body tissues.

ATHEROSCLEROSIS AND HEART DISEASE

Recent evidence demonstrated the prevalence of inflammation in the causal relationship of atherosclerosis to heart disease.[5,6,15,36,38,57,77,83,98] Atherosclerotic plaque may initially form from injury to the endothelial cells within the coronary artery walls. Injury may be initiated by high blood pressure, elevated blood fat levels, and cigarette smoke components (Figure 9.6).[36,83] The current concept of atherosclerotic formation originates with the circulation of white blood cells, namely monocytes, which infiltrate an injured portion of the endothelial wall (Figure 9.7)[15,57,77,83] Within the wall, monocytes convert to macrophages and absorb circulating low-density-lipoprotein cholesterol which has been oxidized and damaged by free-radical modification processes.[7] The engorged macrophages filled with atherogenic cholesterol become generated foam cells at this point. Alternately, platelets become attached to the foam cells and release a platelet-derived growth factor which activates smooth muscle cell proliferation and plaque formation at the site covered by a fibrous cap. The newly formed cap may shear, spewing the atherogenic materials into the bloodstream and forming a thrombotic clot.[57,97,98]

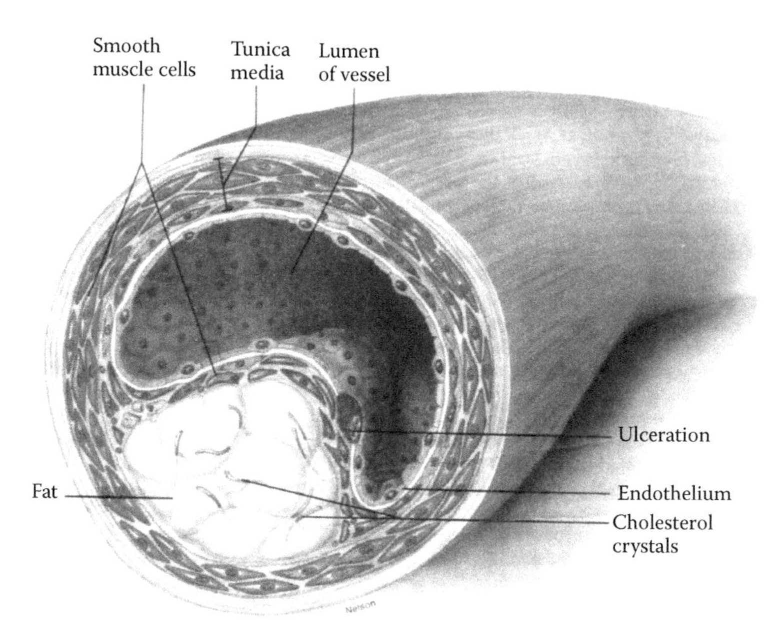

FIGURE 9.6 Atherosclerosis: plaque structure. (From Fox, S.I. *Human Physiology,* W.C. Brown Publishers, New York, 1990. Reproduced with the permission of the McGraw-Hill Companies.)

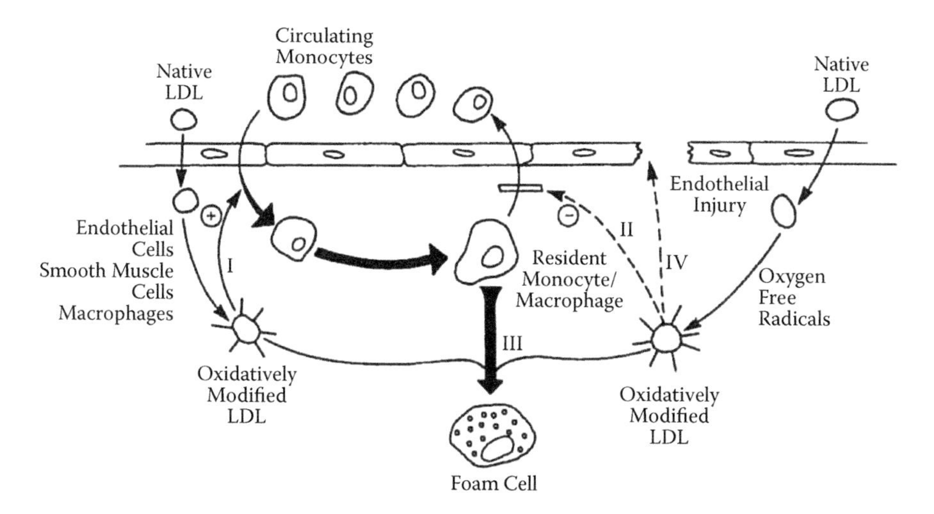

FIGURE 9.7 Concept of atherosclerotic formation. (From Quinn, M.T. et al., *Proceedings National Academy of Sciences USA,* 84, 2995–2998, May, 1987. With permission.)

The causal relationship of blood cholesterol to atherosclerosis and heart disease has been significantly established through epidemiological and biochemical studies. The epidemiological evidence can be demonstrated by review of representative studies in this field of research. The Western Electric Study,[87] a 20-year investigation on dietary cholesterol and heart disease, was conducted in Chicago and involved 1900 middle-aged men. The study included an initial evaluation of dietary food intake, with a follow-up on the same subjects 20 years later. The results demonstrated that those who had consumed higher amounts of saturated fats and cholesterol foods suffered more heart disease deaths than did those who ate lesser amounts of these foods.

The Zutphen Study,[49] a 10-year investigation on the effects of fiber intake and coronary heart disease, was conducted in the Netherlands and included 871 middle-aged men. Mortality from coronary heart disease was almost four times greater for those men who consumed little fiber than for those who had eaten the greatest amount of high-fiber foods.

The Leiden Intervention Study,[6] a 4-year investigation on the relationship between diet, serum lipoproteins, and coronary lesions, was conducted in Leiden and included subjects with one blood vessel obstruction (50%). Food intervention included a 2-year vegetarian diet. The results demonstrated that low-fat dietary intake was of value in preventing the progression of coronary artery disease.

The Ireland–Boston Diet–Heart Study,[52] a 20-year investigation of diet and mortality from heart disease, was conducted in Boston and included 1001 middle-aged men. Mortality from coronary heart disease was higher in those men who consumed greater amounts of saturated fat and cholesterol foods than those who ate more fiber, vegetables, grains, and protein foods.

The Oslo Study Diet and Antismoking Trial,[39] a 5-year study on diet and heart disease, was conducted in Oslo and included 1232 high-risk subjects. The results showed that cholesterol levels were reduced through the intake of a high-polyunsaturated-fat diet and through a reduction in smoking.

The Lipid Research Clinics Coronary Primary Prevention Trials I and II,[50,88,89] a 7- to 10-year investigation of cholesterol reduction through diet and/or drug regimens in relation to coronary heart disease was conducted in the U.S. (12 medical centers) and included 3806 men aged 35 to 59. They had no heart disease, but did have high levels of cholesterol (265 mg/dl of blood and above). All of the subjects consumed low-fat and low-cholesterol foods. Half of these subjects were also treated with cholestyramine, a resin drug that reduced cholesterol levels, while the other dieters received placebos. The results demonstrated that those men who were on a diet alone reduced their cholesterol levels about 4%, while the diet/drug group decreased their levels by 18 to 25%.

The Lifestyle Heart Trial,[70] wherein lifestyle changes were made relative to the adoption of a vegetarian diet providing only 10% of the calories from fat, was conducted on coronary artery diseased patients. The subjects in the study also exercised moderately aerobically, stopped smoking, and practiced stress management. The results showed decreases in both total cholesterol and LDL cholesterol (24.3 and 37%, respectively). HDL cholesterol did not change significantly. The results also showed significant regression in plaque formation.

The Lyon Diet Heart Study[20] a two-and-a-half-year investigation involving 605 men and women, was designed to test whether diet could reduce the chances of a second heart attack occurrence. Half of the participants followed the American Heart Association Step One Diet, while the other half followed the Mediterranean Diet. Originally, the study was scheduled for 5 years but was suspended early after 27 months. The significant results relative to the efficacy of the Mediterranean Diet prompted the decision. The results showed a significant decrease in heart disease–related deaths.

A Mediterranean Style Diet[23] investigation, a 3-month study on cardiovascular risk factor reduction, included 772 adult participants. They were divided into three groups, low fat, Mediterranean Diet with added nut intake, and Mediterranean Diet with added olive oil intake. The comparative results showed that the two Mediterranean Diet groups were more effective in decreasing their blood pressure, blood sugar, and blood lipid levels in contrast to the low fat group.

The biochemical evidence in this frame of reference involves the study of the nature, synthesis, transportation, and utilization of cholesterol in the body relative to the formation of atherosclerotic plaques within the coronary blood vessel walls. Oxidized LDL cholesterol has been identified as the main contributor to this plaque formation.[35] Blood levels of LDL cholesterol are determined by the amount that can be extracted from the blood by cell receptors in the liver.[12] The LDL cholesterol is taken in, broken down, and utilized for cellular purposes relative to cholesterol needs. When such cellular needs are low, excess blood LDL cholesterol accumulates, body cells manufacture few receptors, and little of this blood lipid is taken in for use. When cellular needs are increased, more receptors are made, and more LDL cholesterol is taken in. In this process, however, cellular absorption and use may be critical, since the LDL cholesterol left in the bloodstream, not utilized by the cells, may be oxidized and form plaque within coronary blood vessel walls.[33]

Apoproteins or apolipoproteins have also been studied relative to cholesterol level and the development of atherosclerosis.[53] Apoproteins form the coated lipoprotein complexes that carry triglycerides and cholesterol through the blood. Apoproteins A and C-3 are related to the transportation of HDLs, while apoprotein B is a carrier of LDLs. Triglycerides and VLDLs are transported by apoproteins B and E. The relationship of these apoproteins to the blood lipids they carry may differ relative to atherogenic risk potential.[56]

CHOLESTEROL REDUCTION: NUTRITIONAL INTERVENTION

Fats, carbohydrates, proteins, vitamins, and minerals have been studied relative to cholesterol reduction. Studies have shown that decreases in total fat, saturated fat, and trans fats have reduced total cholesterol levels.[25,57] Monounsaturated and polyunsaturated fats have also been found to decrease cholesterol levels when used in increased ratio amounts or in place of saturated fat.[1,30,36,57] In reference to cholesterol, a reduced intake will result in a lowered serum level.[99] Dietary fats are also involved in the production of prostaglandins and, in this regard, can be of influence in the process of blood platelet aggregation and possible thrombosis.[46,53] In this process, dietary linoleic acid is converted to arachidonic acid, one of the precursors to prostaglandins, and incorporated into platelet membrane phospholipids where it may interact with thromboxane A_1,a platelet aggregating agent, and prostaglandin I_2 and I_3, inhibitors of platelet aggregation.[53] The proportional amounts produced of these agents could determine the degree of platelet aggregation relative to blood clotting processes. Recent studies have shown onions, garlic, and fatty fish to decrease platelet aggregation and promote antiatherosclerotic effects.[18,96] Both onions and garlic are foods from the Allium family and contain similar properties that inhibit thromboxane synthesis and subsequent platelet aggregation. In regard to fatty fish, polyunsaturated omega-3 fatty acids eicosapentaenoic acid (EPA) and docosahexaenoic acid (DHA) have similarly inhibited platelet aggregation.[26] Fatty fish high in EPA and DHA include salmon, mackerel, sablefish, herring, trout, and whitefish. Fish and fatty fish (one meal per week) have also been found to decrease the risk of sudden cardiac death.[26,48]

Carbohydrates have been found to generally raise plasma triglyceride and VLDL levels and to lower HDL levels.[36,84] These effects can be minimized if more complex carbohydrates are ingested. High fiber intakes have been related to decreased levels of cholesterol. Dietary fiber has been classified as soluble and insoluble. The soluble fibers, gums and pectin found in fruit, legumes, and vegetables, have a bile acid cholesterol sequestering or binding ability, which results in a lowering of cholesterol levels.[32,99]

In reference to the effect of protein ingestion upon cholesterol levels, studies have shown that soy, a vegetable protein, is related to the lowering of the serum lipids.[42,84,98] High animal protein intake has been related to an increase in serum cholesterol and triglycerides because of its saturated fat content.

The effects of vitamins and minerals on cholesterol have also been studied.[62] In reference to vitamins, niacin and vitamin C have been found to be of value in this regard. High niacin intake has been related to cholesterol reduction, while a vitamin C deficiency in the body has been found to raise cholesterol levels.[15] The antioxidant properties of vitamins C and E have also been associated with decreased heart disease risk.[20,27] Antioxidants bind to free radicals and neutralize their oxidative damage effects on LDLs.[40] This, in effect, would decrease the amount of circulating oxidized LDL and reduce the proliferation of plaque formation. However, recent evidence has negated these positive relationships. Results from studies have shown that vitamins C and E may have little effect on the oxidation of LDL and may well increase the process of oxidation.[82] Deficiencies of the B vitamins folate, pyridoxine, and cobalamin have also been related to the development of hyperhomocysteinemia, a condition wherein methionine (an amino acid) is converted to homocysteine (a sulfur-based amino acid).[37] High levels of plasma homocysteine can promote and contribute to the development of atherosclerosis through its potential to cause oxidative damage to coronary artery endothelial cells and the development of atherothrombosis.[29] A conditional reversal to methionine can be affected through an increased intake of folate, pyridoxine, and cobalamin, which serve as chemical cofactors in the process. Research has recently found increased homocysteine levels to be of moderate risk.[20] Minerals have also played a significant role in the development of atherosclerosis.[19] Optimal intakes of calcium, sodium, magnesium, chromium, copper, zinc, and iodine can reduce cholesterol risk factors.[99]

DIETARY GOALS AND DIETARY GUIDELINES

In 1977 and 1980, the Senate Select Committee on Nutrition and Human Needs[80] and the Departments of Agriculture and Health, Education, and Welfare,[69] respectively, published position papers on dietary goals and guidelines in an effort to establish a national nutrition policy. Americans at that time were ingesting too much saturated and total fat, too many simple carbohydrates, too much salt, and too many high-cholesterol foods. The established dietary goals included: a reduction in fat from 42 to 30%, no change in protein intake (12 %), and an increase in carbohydrates from 46 to 58%.[80] By 1984, total fat intake had decreased to 36%, with a reduction in saturated fat and an increase in polyunsaturated fat.[78] The dietary guidelines established in 1980 have been revised every 5 years to provide current applicative information relative to nutrient needs.[54,68,92,93,95] Americans were encouraged to consume a variety of foods, to exercise in order to control weight, to increase their intake of grains, vegetables, and fruit, to decrease the amount of fat, saturated fat, cholesterol, salt, and sugar, and to moderate their alcohol intake. In addition, the American Heart Association established guidelines for the daily intake of cholesterol and sodium to 100 mg per 1000 calories (not to exceed 300 mg per day) and 1000 mg per 1000 calories (not to exceed 3000 mg per day), respectively.[1–4,26]

To support these guidelines, food guides and dietary plans were developed and recommended so that nutrient needs could be met on a daily basis. The Pyramid Food Guide divided food intake into five groups: (1) grain, (2) vegetable, (3) fruit, (4) milk, and (5) meat.[94] These groups were presented in the form of numbers of servings per day. Portion sizes and exchanges were included. Grains, vegetables, and fruit were placed in the base of the pyramid, indicating a greater number of servings, while the milk and meat groups were found in the top half, signifying fewer number of servings. At the top of the pyramid fats, oils, and sweets were depicted, to indicate the least amount of servings and to be used sparingly. For those adults with high cholesterol levels, Step One and Step Two Dietary Guidelines were also formulated.[53,64,65,84] The Step One Diet limited saturated fat to less than 10% and cholesterol to less than 300 mg per day. The Step Two Diet limited saturated fat to less than 7% and cholesterol to less than 200 mg per day. Carbohydrate and protein levels were set at 50 to 60% and up to 20%, respectively. However, with the increasing evidential rates of weight gain and obesity over the following years in children and adults, these goals and guidelines were subsequently revised as results of studies demonstrating the changing nature of dietary theory and practice became apparent.[26]

The new dietary goals published in 2002 by the Institute of Medicine reflected these changes based on years of scientific study (Figure A6.2 and Figure A6.3 in Appendix 6).[26] The new goals proposed discretionary ranges in adult calorie intake for carbohydrates from 45 to 65%, fats from 20 to 35%, and protein from 10 to 35%. Daily physical activity was increased from 30 minutes to 60 minutes for cardiovascular health and weight regulation. The intake of fiber was also increased, and recommendations for a decreased intake of total fat, saturated fat, trans fat, and cholesterol were proposed.

The new dietary guidelines published by the United States Department of Agriculture in 2005 generally recommended (Figure A6.4 in Appendix 6):[96]

1. Adequate nutrients within calorie needs — the intake of a variety of nutrient dense foods and the adoption of balanced eating patterns
2. Physical activity and weight management — maintenance of a healthy body weight through an increased amount of physical activity
3. Food groups to encourage — the encouraged consumption of adequate amounts of grains, vegetables, and fruit
4. Fats — the consumption of adequate amounts of monounsaturated and polyunsaturated fats while limiting saturated, trans fat, and cholesterol intake
5. Carbohydrates — the consumption of increased amounts of complex carbohydrates
6. Sodium and potassium — moderated intake of salt and consumption of potassium rich vegetables and fruit
7. Alcoholic beverages — the moderated intake of alcohol

The new food pyramid was revised to support the revised goals and guidelines (Figure 9.8).[25,61,96] The new design was centered in triangular colored bands and

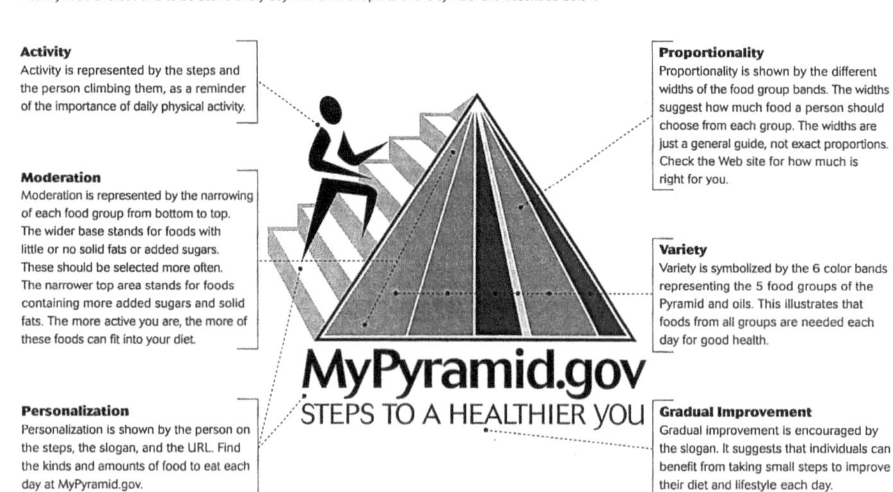

FIGURE 9.8 My pyramid. (From *Dietary Guidelines for Americans 2005*, 6th ed., United States Department of Agriculture, Center for Nutrition Policy and Promotion, April, 2005.)

ascending figure demonstrative of individualized discretionary caloric intake, age level, and physical activity.[13,26,96] The bands denoted the food groups, which included grains, vegetables, fruit, milk, meat, and beans (Figure 9.9). Two food patterns were recommended, namely the Dash Diet (Dietary Approaches to Stop Hypertension) and the USDA (United States Department of Agriculture) Food Guide (Figure 9.10).[96] Both plans were designed to implement eating patterns based on caloric ranges that were demonstrative of the dietary recommendations and based on the increased intake of fruit, vegetables, legumes, whole grains, fish, and low-fat dairy products and a decrease in saturated and hydrogenated fats.[7] In reference to the Dash Diet, nutritional research has demonstrated the healthfulness of the diet relative to disease conditions.[7,31] Probably, one of the more effective diets prevalent today is the Mediterranean Diet. The bulk of the diet includes mostly pasta, grains, vegetables, fruit, yogurt, and olive oil to be consumed daily.[61,98] Sweets, eggs, poultry, and fish are to be eaten a few times per week, and beef intake is restricted to a few times per month. Exercise is mandated, and a glass of wine on a daily basis is encouraged.

Similarly, the American Heart Association has also issued new dietary guidelines.[5,58] Generally, the recommendations include the maintenance of a healthy food intake relative to variety, the maintenance of a healthy body weight relative to physical activity, and the maintenance of desirable blood pressure and blood cholesterol levels relative to healthy eating patterns.

CHOLESTEROL: NORM LEVELS AND RISK ASSESSMENT

A recent review study conducted by the American Heart Association and the National Heart, Lung, and Blood Institute on the relationship of dietary fat to atherosclerosis and heart disease has resulted in newly established blood cholesterol norms (Figure 9.11).[1,2,40,43,66] Desirable blood cholesterol levels for adults have been set at less than 200 milligrams per deciliter of blood (mg/dl), borderline-high levels at 200 to 239 mg/dl, and high levels equal to or greater than 240 mg/dl. Norm range levels for LDL levels were also established. Optimal LDL cholesterol levels were set at less than 100 mg/dl, near optimal at 100–129 mg/dl, borderline-high risk levels at 130 to 159 mg/dl, and high risk levels equal to or greater than 160 mg/dl. Desirable HDL norms were set at levels greater than 40 mg/dl.[79] In reference to heart disease risk assessment, low levels of LDLs and high levels of HDLs are indicated.[86] A further assessment test that may possibly be the most significant in this regard is the ratio of total cholesterol to HDL.[77] Indices of 5.0 for men and 4.4 for women have been established as norm levels. Indices of 3.4 and 3.3 for men and women, respectively, constitute one half the average risk, while indices of 9.6 and 7.1 double the average risk for heart disease.

Blood lipid and lipoprotein levels differ between men and women. Men generally exhibit higher cholesterol, triglyceride, and LDL levels, while women demonstrate higher HDLs and lower cholesterol/HDL ratios than do men.[2]

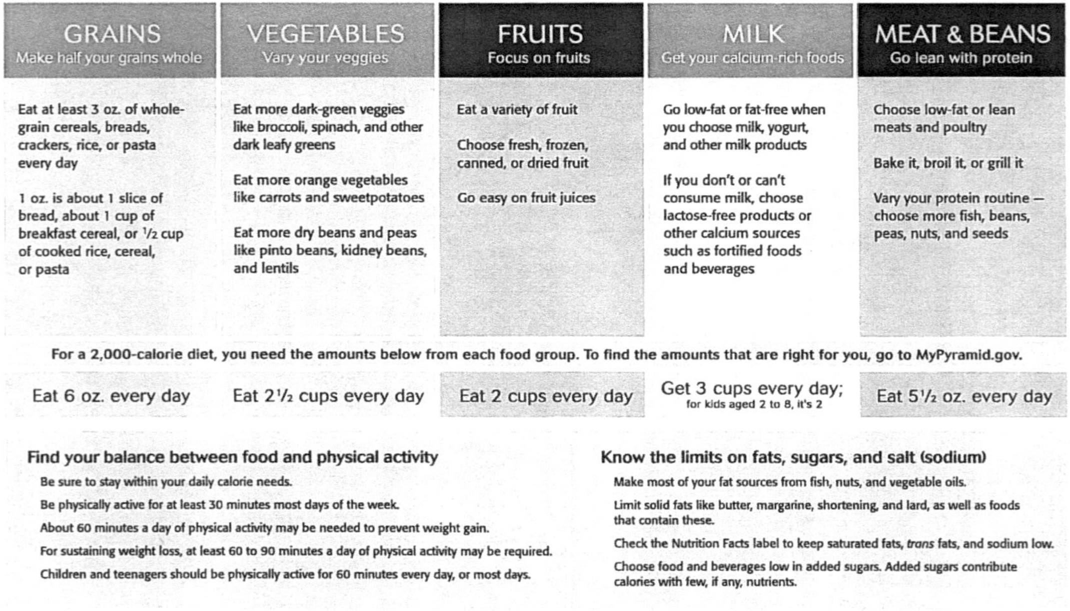

GRAINS Make half your grains whole	VEGETABLES Vary your veggies	FRUITS Focus on fruits	MILK Get your calcium-rich foods	MEAT & BEANS Go lean with protein
Eat at least 3 oz. of whole-grain cereals, breads, crackers, rice, or pasta every day 1 oz. is about 1 slice of bread, about 1 cup of breakfast cereal, or 1/2 cup of cooked rice, cereal, or pasta	Eat more dark-green veggies like broccoli, spinach, and other dark leafy greens Eat more orange vegetables like carrots and sweetpotatoes Eat more dry beans and peas like pinto beans, kidney beans, and lentils	Eat a variety of fruit Choose fresh, frozen, canned, or dried fruit Go easy on fruit juices	Go low-fat or fat-free when you choose milk, yogurt, and other milk products If you don't or can't consume milk, choose lactose-free products or other calcium sources such as fortified foods and beverages	Choose low-fat or lean meats and poultry Bake it, broil it, or grill it Vary your protein routine — choose more fish, beans, peas, nuts, and seeds
For a 2,000-calorie diet, you need the amounts below from each food group. To find the amounts that are right for you, go to MyPyramid.gov.				
Eat 6 oz. every day	Eat 2 1/2 cups every day	Eat 2 cups every day	Get 3 cups every day; for kids aged 2 to 8, it's 2	Eat 5 1/2 oz. every day

Find your balance between food and physical activity

Be sure to stay within your daily calorie needs.

Be physically active for at least 30 minutes most days of the week.

About 60 minutes a day of physical activity may be needed to prevent weight gain.

For sustaining weight loss, at least 60 to 90 minutes a day of physical activity may be required.

Children and teenagers should be physically active for 60 minutes every day, or most days.

Know the limits on fats, sugars, and salt (sodium)

Make most of your fat sources from fish, nuts, and vegetable oils.

Limit solid fats like butter, margarine, shortening, and lard, as well as foods that contain these.

Check the Nutrition Facts label to keep saturated fats, *trans* fats, and sodium low.

Choose food and beverages low in added sugars. Added sugars contribute calories with few, if any, nutrients.

FIGURE 9.9 My pyramid food groups. (From *Dietary Guidelines for Americans 2005,* 6th ed., United States Department of Agriculture, Center for Nutrition Policy and Promotion, April, 2005.)

The USDA Food Guide and The Dash Eating Plan at the 2,000 Calorie Level Figure

Food Groups and Subgroups	USDA Food Guide Amount[b]	DASH Eating Plan Amount	Equivalent Amounts
Fruit Group	2 cups (4 servings)	2 to 2.5 cups (4 to 5 servings)	1/2 cup is equivalent is: • 1/2 cup fresh, frozen, or canned fruit • 1 med fruit • 1/4 cup dried fruit • 1/2 cup fruit juice
Vegetable Group	2.5 cups (5 servings)	2 to 2.5 cups (4 to 5 servings)	1/2 cup equivalent is: • 1/2 cup of cut-up raw or cooked vegetable • 1 cup raw leafy vegetable • 1/2 cup vegetable juice
• Dark green vegetables	3 cups/week		
• Orange vegetables	2 cups/week		
• Legumes (dry beans)	3 cups/week		
• Starchy vegetables	3 cups/week		
• Other vegetables	6.5 cups/week		
Grain Group	6 ounce-equivalents	6 to 8 ounce-equivalents (6 to 8 servings)	1 ounce-equivalent is: • 1 slice bread • 1 cup dry cereal • 1/2 cup cooked rice, pasta, cereal • DASH: 1 oz dry cereal (1/2–1 1/4 cup depending on creal type — check label)
• Whole grains	3 ounce-equivalents		
• Other grains	3 ounce-equivalents		
Meat and Beans Group	5.5 ounce-equivalents	6 ounces or less meat, poultry, fish 4 to 5 servings per week nuts, seeds, and legumes[d]	1 ounce-equivalent is: • 1 ounce of cooked lean meats, poultry, fish • 1 egg • USDA: 1/4 cup cooked dry beans or tofu, 1 Tbsp peanut butter, 1/2 oz nuts or seeds • DASH: 1 1/2 oz nuts, 2 Tbsp peanut butter, 1/2 oz seeds, 1/2 cup cooked dry beans
Milk Group	3 cups	2 to 3 cups	1 cup equivalent is: • 1 cup low-fat/fat-free milk, yogurt • 1 1/2 oz of low-fat, fat-free or reduced fat natural cheese • 2 oz of low-fat or fat-free processed cheese
Oils	27 grams (6 tsp)	8 to 12 grams (2 to 3 tsp)	DASH: 1 tsp equivalent is: • 1 tsp soft margarine • 1 Tsp low-fat mayo • 2 Tbsp light salad dressing • 1 tsp vegetable oil
Discretionary Calorie Allowance			DASH: 1 Tsp added sugar equivalent is:
• Example of distribution	267 calories		• 1 Tbsp jelly or jam
Solid fat	18 grams		• 1/2 cup sorbet and ices
Added sugars	8 tsp	~2 tsp (5 Tbsp per week)	• 1 cup lemonade

Note: Amounts of various food groups that are recommended each day or each week in the USDA Food Guide and in the DASH Eating Plan (amounts are daily unless otherwise specified) at the 2,000-calorie level. Also identified are equivalent amounts for different food choices in each group. To follow either eating pattern, food choices over time should provide these amounts of food from each group on average.

[a]All servings are per day unless otherwise noted. USDA vegetable subgroup amounts and amounts of DASH nuts, seeds, and dry beans are per week. [b]The 2,000-calorie USDA Food Guide is appropriate for many sedentary males 51 to 70 years of age, sedentary females 19 to 30 years of age, and for some other gender/age groups who are more physically active. See table 3 for information about gender/age/activity levels and appropriate calorie intakes. See appendices A-2 and A-3 for more information on the food groups, amounts, and food intake patterns at other calorie levels. [c]Whole grains are recommended for most grain servings to meet fiber recommendations. [d]In the DASH Eating Plan, nuts, seeds, and legumes are a separate food group from eats, poultry, and fish. [e]Since eggs are high in cholestrol, limit egg yolk intake to no more than 4 per week; 2 egg whites have the same protein content as 1 oz of meat. [f]The oils listed in this table are considered to be part of discretionary calories because they are a major source of the vitamin E and polyunsaturated fatty acids, including the essential fatty acids in the food pattern. In contrast, solid fats (i.e., saturated and trans fat) are listed separately as a source of discretionary calories.

FIGURE 9.10 The USDA food guide and the Dash Eating Plan at the 2,000-Calorie level figure. (From *Dietary Guidelines for Americans 2005,* 6th ed., United States Department of Agriculture. Center for Nutrition Policy and Promotion, April, 2005.)

Cholesterol Classifications

Total Cholesterol	
Less than 200 mg/dL	Desirable
200-239 mg/dL	Borderline high
240 mg/dL and above	High
LDL Cholesterol	
Less than 100 mg/dL	Optimal (ideal)
100-129 mg/dL	Near optimal/above optimal
130-159 mg/dL	Borderline high
160-189 mg/dL	High
190 mg/dL and above	Very high
HDL Cholesterol	
Less than 40 mg/dL	Major heart disease risk factor
60 mg/dL and above	Gives some protection against heart disease

FIGURE 9.11 Cholesterol classifications. (From Your Guide to Lowering Your Cholesterol With TLC. National Institutes of Health. National Heart, Lung, and Blood Institute. NIH Publication No. 06-5235, December, 2005.)

MAJOR RISK FACTORS

Related risk factors to those of blood lipids and lipoproteins include [64,65,85]

age	hypertension
gender	obesity
heredity	physical inactivity
dyslipidemia	cigarette smoking

In reference to age, the process itself indicates that as people age, the development of coronary heart disease may become more prevalent, because of the body's failure and ability to regulate the absorption, synthesis, and excretion of lipids.[85] In reference to gender, heart disease rate for women is lower than that for men and is demonstrated by longer life expectancy figures. Hormonal factors may partly account for such differences. Estrogen levels in premenopausal women are high and have been related to lower heart disease rates, while testosterone hormone levels in men are related to possible disease development.[34] Women also have higher HDL levels than do men.[53] Recent study in this area indicates that higher levels of this lipoprotein lessen the risk for heart disease. Heredity may also be of influence relative to heart disease risk. Familial high blood lipid levels may be inherited and may account for early development of heart disease symptoms.[53,98] Biochemical mechanism failure may be a determining factor relative to the absorption and utilization of cholesterol and triglycerides.[12]

High serum lipids have been found to be related to increased heart disease risk.[16] In reference to cholesterol, LDLs play a primary role in the atherogenic process, while HDLs have been found to be inversely related to this process and judged to be more protective in nature.[29] High triglyceride levels have also been reported to be related to coronary heart disease risk.[53,91] Recent studies have found high triglyceride levels to be an independent risk factor.[91] Triglycerides levels may also be related to high VLDL and LDL levels, which may be indicative of an increased heart disease risk.[36,53,95]

Cigarette smoking has been classified as one of the major risk factors to the development of heart disease.[41,60] Smoking increases levels of plasma triglycerides and VLDLs and decreases levels of HDLs.[29] Its effects may also be long term, due to chronic endothelium hypoxia and platelet alteration, which may promote the process of atherosclerosis.[44,75] In this regard, the number of years and the number of cigarettes smoked over a lifetime may be related to the severity of coronary artery disease.[76] Smoking is accountable for 20% of heart disease–related deaths.[98]

Hypertension or high blood pressure is another of the major risk factors (Figure 9.12).[66,90] Recent National Health and Nutrition Examination Survey results estimate that 24% (43 million) of the adult men and women in this country suffer from high blood pressure.[47] Increased levels of systolic and/or diastolic blood pressure have been associated with the risk of coronary heart disease.[17,90] The eventual high pressure may weaken the arterial walls and result in injury to blood vessels.[29]

Obesity has been implicated as a risk factor in the development of atherosclerosis and heart disease.[35,57] Excess weight has been reported to be significantly related to high serum cholesterol levels.[66] Glueck[32] found excess weight and obesity to be related to high triglyceride and low HDL levels in both men and women. Similar results were also obtained by Garrison et al.[30] relative to obesity and high LDL levels and high cholesterol–HDL ratio indices. Results from the 1979 Build Study[67] have indicated that mortality risks relative to heart disease were greatest for those in the extreme overweight and underweight categories. Recent evidence in this area of study has shown that body fat location can be a factor in heart disease risk. Increased abdominal circumference and android waist/hip ratio measures have been related to a higher risk in this regard.[87,91,102] A National Health and Nutrition Examination Survey recently found that the prevalence of obesity in the U.S. has been steadily increasing and may result in a greater risk of morbidity and mortality.[51,60]

In reference to physical inactivity, recent studies have shown that exercise may be of benefit in the reduction of triglycerides, VLDLs, and LDLs, and in the increase of HDLs.[53,72] Studies of San Francisco longshoremen and Harvard University alumni have also demonstrated the evidential relationship between inactivity, exercise, and heart disease.[55,61,71,73] In a study of 2907 active men and women relative to cardiovascular fitness and heart disease risk, Bovens et al.[11] found that the more fit subjects exhibited significantly lower risk. These results were corroborated by Ekelund et al.[22] and Blair et al.[8–10] The Heritage Family Study on fitness and fatness found both

Blood Pressure Levels for Adults*

Category	Systolic† (mmHg)‡		Diastolic† (mmHg)‡	Result
Normal	Less than 120	*and*	Less than 80	Good for you!
Prehypertension	120-139	*or*	80-89	Your blood pressure could be a problem. Make changes in what you eat and drink, be physically active, and lose extra weight. If you also have diabetes, see your doctor.
Hypertension	140 or higher	*or*	90 or higher	You have high blood pressure. Ask your doctor or nurse how to control it.

* *For adults ages 18 and older who are not on medicine for high blood pressure and do not have a short-term serious illness. Source:* The Seventh Report of the Joint National Committee on Prevention, Detection, Evaluation, and Treatment of High Blood Pressure: *NIH Publication No. 03-5230, National High Blood Pressure Education Program, May 2003.*

† *If systolic and diastolic pressures fall into different categories, overall status is the higher category.*

‡ *Millimeters of mercury.*

FIGURE 9.12 Blood pressure levels for adults. (From Your Guide to Lowering Your Blood Pressure With Dash. National Institutes of Health. National Heart, Lung, and Blood Institute. NIH Publication No. 06-4082, April, 2006.)

obesity and physical inactivity to be risk predictors.[45] Similarly, the Honolulu Heart and the Ten Thousand Step Programs, wherein walking was used as the exercise criteria, were also demonstrated a decrease in heart disease risk.[37,101] The influence of exercise upon the risk factors of obesity, high blood pressure, and blood lipids and lipoproteins has also been beneficial toward the promotion of overall health and decreased all-cause mortality (Figure 9.13).[10,14,21,34,36,53,58,59,64,72,74]

THE METABOLIC SYNDROME

In addition to these major risk factors, there is also the metabolic syndrome, a cluster of conditions related to heart disease, diabetes, and mortality (Figure 9.14). The results of the Third National Health and Nutrition Examination Survey identified and denoted the prevalence of the related components.[27,28] Abdominal obesity, atherogenic dyslipidemia, high blood pressure, and insulin resistance are conditions which

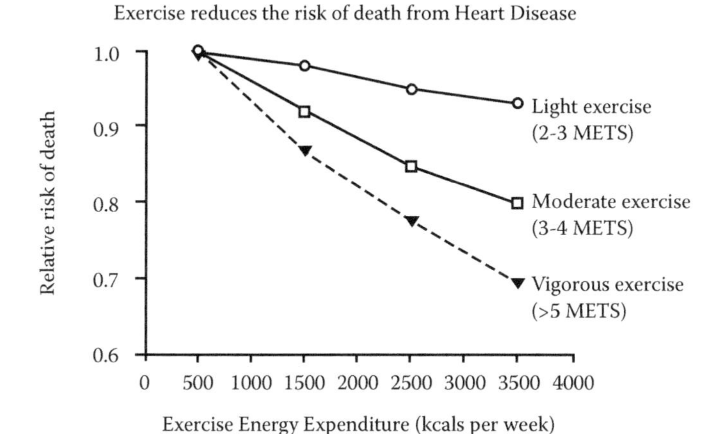

1 MET = Energy expended while resting

3-4 METs = Energy expended while walking very fast

5-6 METs = Energy expended during slow running

FIGURE 9.13 Exercise intensity and risk of heart disease. (From Powers, S.K. Exercise, Antioxidants, and Cardioprotection. Gatorade Sports Science Exchange, The Gatorade Sports Science Institute, 15, No. 2, 2002. With permission.)

are indicative of the prevalence of prothrombotic and inflammatory increased risks for heart disease.[24,79,91]

BIOCHEMICAL RISK FACTORS

Prominent and associated risk factors that are considered to be inflammatory markers include high sensitivity C-reactive protein, high homocysteine, and high fibrinogen levels.[29,64,103] C-reactive protein levels reflect an inflammatory relationship to endothelial dysfunction, atherosclerotic plaque, and the possibility of plaque rupture. High homocysteine levels indicate an increased endothelial dysfunction as well as platelet aggregation risk for ischemic heart disease, stroke, and peripheral vascular disease. In regard to high fibrinogen levels, the risk is related to coagulant blood properties and increased fibrin accumulation.

SUMMARY

In summary, the relationship of nutrition to the development of atherosclerosis and heart disease has been substantially investigated. Research results have generally shown that:

1. The major lipid components in blood are triglycerides, phospholipids, and cholesterol.

Risk Factor	Defining Level
Abdominal Obesity	Waist Circumference†
Men	>102 cm (>40 in)
Women	>88 cm (>35 in)
Triglycerides	≥150 mg/dL
HDL cholesterol	
Men	<40 mg/dL
Women	<50 mg/dL
Blood pressure	≥130/85 mmHg
Fasting glucose	≥110 mg/dL

* The ATP III panel did not find adequate evidence to recommend routine measurement of insulin resistance (e.g., plasma insulin), proinflammatory state (e.g., high-sensitivity C-reactive protein), or prothrombotic state (e.g., fibrinogen or PAI-1) in the diagnosis of the metabolic syndrome.

† Some male persons can develop multiple metabolic risk factors when the waist circumference is only marginally increased, e.g., 94-102 cm (37-39 in). Such persons may have a strong genetic contribution to insulin resistance. They should benefit from changes in life habits, similarly to men with categorical increases in waist circumference.

FIGURE 9.14 Metabolic syndrome risk factors. (From Third Report of the National Cholesterol Education Program (NCEP) Expert Panel on Detection, Evaluation, and Treatment of High Blood Cholesterol in Adults (Adult Treatment Panel III) Final Report. National Institutes of Health. National Heart, Lung, and Blood Institute. NIH Publication No. 02-5215, September, 2002.)

2. There are basically four major types of lipoproteins which are classified according to increasing density, protein, and phospholipid concentrations and decreasing triglyceride levels.
3. Recent evidence has demonstrated the prevalence of inflammation in the causal relationship of atherosclerosis to heart disease.
4. Epidemiological and biochemical studies have significantly established the causal relationship of atherosclerosis to heart disease.
5. Studies have shown that decreases in total fat, saturated fat, cholesterol, simple carbohydrates, and animal protein can result in the lowering of cholesterol levels.
6. Recent evidence has shown that vitamins C and E have little effect on the oxidation of LDL and may well increase the process of oxidation.
7. The biochemical mechanisms of cholesterol synthesis, transportation, and utilization by the body play a significant role in the development of atherosclerosis and heart disease.
8. Dietary goals, dietary guidelines, and dietary food plans for Americans have been established in an effort to promote nutritional health.
9. Blood lipid and lipoprotein norm range levels have been established for both children and adults.

10. There are interactive relationships between age, gender, obesity, cigarette smoking, high blood lipids, hypertension, physical inactivity, and heart disease risk levels.
11. The metabolic syndrome is a cluster of disease condition risk factors that are related to atherosclerosis and heart disease.
12. Inflammatory markers such as high C-reactive protein, high homocysteine, and high fibrinogen levels are considered to be associated risk factors for heart disease.

GLOSSARY

Antioxidants Beta carotene (a precursor to vitamin A) and vitamin E are considered to be antioxidants that have the ability to bind to free radicals and neutralize their oxidative damaging effects on low-density lipoproteins

Apoproteins or apolipoproteins The coated lipoprotein complexes that carry triglycerides and cholesterol through the blood

Atherosclerosis A condition in which fatty substances form plaque inside coronary arteries

Cholesterol A sterol, an essential metabolite, and a fat-like substance

Chylomicrons Lipoproteins that are large in size, light in weight, and contain triglycerides

Cis fatty acids Empty hydrogen bonds formed on one side of the carbon atom

Free radical formation An unpaired oxygen electron that has the ability to oxidize and damage LDL cholesterol

High-density lipoproteins (HDL) Lipoproteins that are small in size, dense in weight, and are the main carriers of cholesterol from the body tissues

Inflammation A biochemical factor that may be prevalent in the formation of plaque in the coronary arteries

Lipoproteins Fat carriers of cholesterol and triglycerides in blood

Low-density lipoproteins (LDL) Lipoproteins that contain mostly cholesterol and are the prime carriers of this sterol to body tissues

Macrophages White blood cells that can engulf oxidized LDL cholesterol and become generated foam cells

Metabolic syndrome A cluster of disease condition risk factors that are interrelated to atherosclerosis and heart disease

Monocytes One of the white blood cells circulating in the blood

Monounsaturated fat Fatty acids in which the carbon chain has a double bond, with two atoms of hydrogen missing

Omega-3 fatty acids Fatty acids found in fatty fish that are high in eicosapentaenoic and docosahexaenoic acids that may inhibit red blood platelet aggregation

Pectin A soluble fiber found in fruit

Phospholipids Fat compounds that contain glycerol, two fatty acids, and one phosphoric acid with a nitrogenous base

Platelet-derived growth factor A factor produced by platelets that activates smooth muscle cell proliferation

Polyunsaturated fat Fatty acids in which the carbon chain has two or more double bonds

Prostaglandin I^2 and I^3 Inhibitors of blood platelet aggregation

Prostaglandins Fatty acids that can regulate blood pressure, blood flow, and the dilation of blood vessels

Saturated fat Fatty acids in which the carbon chain contains a full compliment of hydrogen-filled bonds

Thromboxane A^2 A platelet aggregating agent

Trans fatty acids Fatty acids in which the carbon atoms do not contain a full complement of hydrogen atoms on both sides of the carbon chain.

Triglycerides Fat compounds that contain glycerol and three fatty acids

Type A behavior Competitive, aggressive, and goal-driven personality

Type B behavior Relaxed, calm, and nonpressured personality

Unsaturated fat Fatty acids in which the carbon chain does not contain a full compliment of hydrogen atoms

Very low-density lipoproteins (VLDL) Lipoproteins that are partially degraded chylomicrons and contain mostly triglycerides

REFERENCES

1. American Heart Association and the National Heart, Lung, and Blood Institute, Recommendations Regarding Public Screening for Measuring Blood Cholesterol. NIH Publication No. 95-3045, September, 1995.
2. American Heart Association and the National Heart, Lung, and Blood Institute, The cholesterol facts: a summary of the evidence relating dietary fats, serum cholesterol, and coronary heart disease, *Circulation,* 81, 1721–1733, May 1990.
3. American Heart Association, A statement for health professionals from the Nutrition Committee. *Dietary guidelines for healthy American adults, Circulation,* 94, 1795–1800, 1996.
4. American Heart Association, Dietary guidelines for healthy American adults: a statement for health professionals from the Nutrition Committee, *Circulation,* 94, 1795–1800, 1996.
5. American Heart Association, Dietary Guidelines, Revision 2000: a statement for healthcare professionals from the Nutrition Committee of the American Heart Association, *Circulation,* 102, 2284, 2000.
6. Arnatzenius, A.C. et al., Diet, lipoproteins, and the progression of coronary atherosclerosis: the Leiden Intervention Trial, *New England Journal of Medicine,* 312, 805–811, 1985.
7. Appel, L.J. et al., Effects of protein, monounsaturated fat, and carbohydrate intake on blood pressure and serum lipids. Results of the Omni Heart Randomized Trial, *Journal of the American Medical Association,* 294, 2455–2464, 2005.
8. Blair, S.N. et al., Changes in physical fitness and all-cause mortality. A prospective study of healthy and unhealthy men, *Journal of the American Medical Association,* 278, 1095–1098, 1966.

9. Blair, S.N. et al., Physical fitness and all cause mortality. A prospective study of healthy men and women, *Journal of American Medical Association,* 262, 2395–2401, 1989.
10. Blair, S.N. et al., Influences of cardiorespiratory fitness and other precursors on cardiovascular disease and all-cause mortality in men and women, *Journal of the American Medical Association,* 276, 205–210, 1996.
11. Bovens, A.M. et al., Physical activity, fitness, and selected risk factors for CHDS in active men and women, *Medicine and Science in Sports and Exercise,* 25, 572–576, May, 1993.
12. Brown, M.S., and J.L. Goldstein, How LDL receptors influence cholesterol and atherosclerosis, *Scientific American,* 251, 58–66, 1984.
13. Burke, L M., The I O C Consensus on Sport Nutrition: new guidelines for nutrition for athletes, *International Journal of Sport Nutrition and Exercise Metabolism,* 13, 549–552, 2003.
14. Chambliss, H.O., Exercise duration and intensity in a weight loss program, *Clinical Journal of Sports Medicine,* 15, 113–115, 2005.
15. Collins, J., Monocyte: attracting protein may initiate atherosclerosis, *Research Resources Reporter,* 15, 1–3, September, 1991.
16. Committee on Diet and Health, *Diet and Health: Implications for Reducing Chronic Disease Risk,* National Academy Press, Washington, DC, 1989.
17. Dash Collaborative Research Group, A clinical trial of the effects of dietary patterns on blood pressure, *New England Journal of Medicine,* 336, 1117–1124, 1999.
18. Daviglus, M.L. et al., Fish consumption and the 30-year risk of fatal myocardial infarction, *New England Journal of Medicine,* 336, 1046–1053, 1997.
19. de Lorgeril, M. et al., Mediterranean diet, traditional risk factors and the rate of cardiovascular complications after myocardial infarction: final report of the Lyon Diet Heart Study, *Circulation,* 99, 779–785, 1999.
20. Doll, R. et al., Mortality in relation to smoking: 50 years' observations on male British doctors, *British Medical Journal,* 328, 1519, 2004.
21. Dunn, A.L. et al., Comparison of lifestyle and structured interventions to increase physical activity and cardiorespiratory fitness: a randomized trial, *Journal of the American Medical Association,* 281, 327–334, 1999.
22. Ekelund, L.G. et al., Physical fitness as a predictor of cardiovascular mortality in asymptomatic North American men. The Lipid Research Clinics Mortality Follow-up Study, *New England Journal of Medicine,* 319, 1379, 1988.
23. Estruch, R. et al., Effects of a Mediterranean-style diet on cardiovascular risk factors: a randomized trial, *Annals of Internal Medicine,* 145, 1–11, 2006.
24. Ferreira, I. et al., The metabolic syndrome, cardiopulmonary fitness, and subcutaneous trunk fat as independent determinants of arterial stiffness. The American Growth and Health Longitudinal Study, Archives of Internal Medicine, 165, 875–882, 2005.
25. Fink, H.H., M.S. Burgoon, and A.E. Mikesky, *Practical Applications in Sports Nutrition,* Jones and Bartlett Publishers, Sudbury, MA, 2006.
26. Food and Nutrition Board, Institute of Medicine, *Dietary Reference Intakes for Energy, Carbohydrates, Fiber, Fat, Fatty Acids, Cholesterol, Protein, and Amino Acids,* National Academy Press, Washington, DC, 2002.
27. Ford, E., W.H. Giles, and W.H. Dietz, Prevalence of the metabolic syndrome among U.S. adults: findings from the Third National Health and Nutrition Survey, *Journal of the American Medical Association,* 287, 356–359, 2002.
28. Galbut, B.H. and M.H. Davidson, Practical applications of the NCEP ATP III updates, *Patient Care,* 31–38, March, 2005.

29. Gandhi, H.A. and M.K. Shah, Nonlipid serum markers for clinical risk assessment of coronary artery disease, *Resident and Staff Physician,* 51, 15–24, 2005.
30. Garrison, R.J. et al., Obesity and lipoprotein cholesterol in the Framingham offspring study, *Metabolism,* 29, 1053–1060, 1980.
31. Gifford, K.D., Dietary fats, eating guides, and public policy: history, critique, and recommendations, *American Journal of Medicine,* 113, 89S-106S, December 30, 2002.
32. Glueck, D.J., *Relationships of Age, Sex, Race, Obesity, and Exercise to HDL Epidemiology of Plasma High-Density Lipoprotein Cholesterol Levels: The Lipid Research Clinics Program Prevalence Study,* National Heart, Blood, and Lung Institute, Washington, DC, 1980.
33. Goldstein, J.L., T. Kita, and M.S. Brown, Defective lipoprotein receptors and atherosclerosis, *New England Journal of Medicine,* 309, 288–296, 1983.
34. Gordon, N.F. and L.W. Gibbons, *The Cooper Clinic Cardiac Rehabilitation Program,* Simon and Schuster, New York, 1990.
35. Gordon, T. et al., High density lipoprotein as a protective factor against coronary heart disease: the Framingham Study, *American Journal of Medicine,* 62, 707–714, 1977.
36. Gotto, A. and H. Pownall, *Manual of Lipid Disorders. Reducing the Risk for Coronary Heart Disease,* 3rd ed., Lippincott, Williams, and Wilkins, Philadelphia, 2003.
37. Hakim, A.A. et al., Effects of walking on coronary heart disease in elderly men. The Honolulu Heart Program, *Circulation,* 100, 9–13, 1999.
38. Hansson, G.K., Inflammation, atherosclerosis, and coronary artery disease, *New England Journal of Medicine,* 352, 1685–1695, 2005.
39. Hjermann, I., I. Holme, and P. Leren, Oslo Study Diet and Antismoking Trial Results after 102 months, *American Journal of Medicine,* 10, 7–11, 1986.
40. Hodis, H.N. et al., Serial coronary angiographic evidence that antioxidant vitamin intake reduces progression of coronary artery atherosclerosis, *Journal of the American Medical Association,* 278, 1849–1854, 1995.
41. Howard, G. et al., Cigarette smoking and progression of atherosclerosis: the atherosclerosis risk in communities (ARIC) study, *Journal of the American Medical Association,* 279, 119–124, 1998.
42. Jancin, B., Meta-analysis shows soy supplements reduce serum lipids, *Internal Medicine News,* 38, 6, 2005.
43. Jenkins, D.J.A., C.W.C. Kendall, and A. Marchie, Diet and cholesterol reduction, *Annals of Internal Medicine,* 142, 793–795, 2005.
44. Kannel, W.B., Cigarettes, coronary occlusions, and myocardial infarction, *Journal of the American Medical Association,* 246, 871–872, 1981.
45. Katzmarzyk, P.T. et al., Fitness, fatness, and estimated coronary disease risk: the Heritage Family Study, *Medicine and Science in Sports and Exercise,* 33, 585–590, 2001.
46. Kinsella, J.E. et al., Metabolism of trans fatty acids with emphasis on the effects of trans, trans-octadecadienoate on lipid composition, essential fatty acid, and prostaglandins: an overview, *American Journal of Clinical Nutrition,* 34, 2307–2318, 1981.
47. Landers, S.J., Dietary guide: eat less, exercise more, *American Medical News,* 47, 36, September 13, 2004.
48. Kromhout, D. Fish consumption and sudden cardiac death, *Journal of the American Medical Association,* 279, 65–66, 1988.
49. Kromhout, D., E.B. Bosschuter, and C. DeLezanne Coulander, Dietary fibre and 10-year mortality from coronary heart disease, cancer, and all causes, *Lancet,* 1, 518–521, 1982.

50. Krormal, R.A., Commentary on the published results of the Lipid Research Clinics Coronary Primary Prevention Trial, *Journal of the American Medical Association,* 253, 2091–2093, 1985.
51. Kuczmarski, R.J. et al., Increasing prevalence of overweight among U.S. adults. The National Health and Nutrition Examination Surveys, *Journal of the American Medical Association,* 272, 205–211, July 20, 1994.
52. Kushi, L.H. et al., Diet and 20-year mortality from coronary heart disease. The Ireland-Boston Diet-Heart Study, *New England Journal of Medicine,* 312, 811–818, 1985.
53. Kwiterovich, P.O., *The Johns Hopkins Complete Guide for Preventing and Reversing Heart Disease,* Prima Publishing, Rocklin, CA, 1993.
54. Lawn, R.M., Lipoprotein (a) in heart disease, *Scientific American,* 259, 54–60, June, 1992.
55. Lee, I-Min, C.C. Hsush, and R.S. Paffenbarger, Exercise intensity and longevity in men: the Harvard Alumni Health Study, *Journal of the American Medical Association,* 273, 1179–1184, 1995.
56. Leiden, J.M., Adenovirus-mediated gene transfer as an *in vivo* probe of lipoprotein metabolism, *Circulation,* 94, 2046–2051, 1996.
57. Libby, P., Atherosclerosis: the new view, Scientific American, 379, 47–55, May, 2002.
58. Lichtenstein, A.H. et al., Diet and lifestyle recommendations, Revision 2006. A scientific statement from the American Heart Association Nutrition Committee, *Circulation,* 114, 82–96, 2006.
59. Manson, J.E. et al., Walking compared with vigorous exercise for the prevention of cardiovascular events in women, *New England Journal of Medicine,* 347(10): 716–725, 2002.
60. Mark, D.H., Deaths attributable to obesity, *Journal of the American Medical Association,* 293, 1918, 2005.
61. Mitka, M., Government unveils new food pyramid: critics say nutrition tool is flawed, *Journal of the American Medical Association,* 293, 2581–2582, 2005.
62. Morris, C.D. and S. Carson, Routine vitamin supplementation to prevent cardiovascular disease: a summary of the evidence for the U.S. Preventive Task Force, *Annals of Internal Medicine,* 139, 56–70, 2003.
63. Multiple risk factor intervention trial. Risk factor changes and mortality results, *Journal of the American Medical Association,* 248, 1465–1477, 1982.
64. Nash, D.T., C-reactive protein: a promising new marker of cardiovascular risk? *Consultant,* 45, 453–460, April 1, 2005.
65. National Institutes of Health, National Heart, Lung, and Blood Institute, *The Practical Guide: Identification, Evaluation, and Treatment of Overweight and Obesity in Adults,* National Institutes of Health, National Heart, Lung, and Blood Institute, Bethesda, MD, 2000.
66. Nichols, A.B. et al., Independence of serum lipid levels and dietary habits, The Tecumseh Study, *Journal of the American Medical Association,* 236, 1949–1953, 1976.
67. Society of Actuaries and Association of Life Insurance Medical Directors of America, *1979 Build Study,* Society of Actuaries and Association of Life Insurance Medical Directors of America, Chicago, 1980.
68. *Nutrition and Your Health: Dietary Guidelines for Americans,* The American Medical Association, Chicago, 1980.

69. *Nutrition and Your Health: Dietary Guidelines for Americans,* U.S. Department of Agriculture and of Health, Education, and Welfare, U.S. Government Printing Office, Washington, DC, 1980.
70. Ornish, D. et al., Can life-style changes reverse coronary heart disease? The Life-style Heart Trial, *Lancet,* 336, 129–133, 1990.
71. Paffenbarger, R.S., Jr., and R.T. Hyde, Exercise as protection against a heart attack, *New England Journal of Medicine,* 302, 1026–1027, 1980.
72. Paffenbarger, R.S., Jr. et al., Work energy level, personal characteristics and fatal heart attack: a birth-cohort effect, *American Journal of Epidemiology,* 105, 200–213, 1977.
73. Paffenbarger, R.S., Jr., A.L. Wing, and R.T. Hyde, Physical activity as an index of heart attack risk in college alumni, *American Journal of Epidemiology,* 408, 161–175, 1978.
74. President's Council on Physical Fitness and Sports, Physical activity in the prevention and management of coronary heart disease, *Physical Activity and Fitness Research Digest,* 2, 1–7, 1995.
75. Ramsdale, D.R. et al., Smoking and coronary artery disease assessed by routine coronary arteriography, *British Medical Journal,* 290-:197–200, 1985.
76. Rationale of the diet-heart statement of the American Heart Association, Report of the Nutrition Committee, *Circulation,* 88, 3008–3029, December, 1993.
77. Rethinking Cholesterol, *Harvard Health Letter,* 17, 6–8, June, 1992.
78. Rifkind, B.M., Cholesterol redux, *Journal of the American Medical Association,* 264, 3060–3061, December 19, 1990.
79. Ross, R. and I. Jansson, Is abdominal fat preferentially reduced in response to exercise-induced weight loss? *Medicine and Science in Sports and Exercise,* 257, S568–S572, 1999.
80. Select Committee on Nutrition and Human Needs, U.S. Senate, *Dietary Goals for the United States,* 2nd ed., U.S. Government Printing Office, Washington, DC, 1977.
81. Shekelle, R.B. et al., Diet, serum cholesterol, and death from coronary heart disease: the Western Electric Study, *New England Journal of Medicine,* 304, 64–69, 1981.
82. Shishehbor, M.H. and S.L. Hazen, Antioxidant studies need a change of direction, *Cleveland Clinic Journal of Medicine,* 71, 285–288,2004.
83. Steinberg, D. and J.L. Witztum, Lipoproteins and atherogenesis: current concepts, *Journal of the American Medical Association,* 264, 3047–3052, December 19, 1990.
84. Stone, N.J. et al., Summary of the scientific conference on the efficacy of hypocho-lesterolemic dietary interventions, *Circulation,* 94, 3388–3391, 1996.
85. Summary of the second report of the National Cholesterol Education Program (NCEP) Expert Panel on Detection, Evaluation and Treatment of High Blood Cholesterol in Adults (Adult Treatment Panel II). *Journal of the American Medical Association,* 269, 3015–3023, 1993.
86. The European Concerted Action Project, Plasma homocysteine as a risk factor for vascular disease, *Journal of the American Medical Association,* 277, 1776–1781, 1997.
87. The Institute of Food Technologists Expert panel on Food, Safety and Nutrition, Human obesity, *Contemporary Nutrition,* 18, 1–4, 1993.
88. The Lipid Research Clinics Coronary Primary Prevention Trial result I. Reduction in incidence of coronary heart disease, *Journal of the American Medical Association,* 251, 351–364, 1984.

89. The Lipid Research Clinics Coronary Primary Prevention Trial results II. The relationship of reduction in incidence of coronary heart disease to cholesterol lowering, *Journal of the American Medical Association,* 251, 365–374, 1984.
90. National High Blood Pressure Education Program, The Seventh Report of the Joint National Committee on Prevention, Detection, Evaluation, and Treatment of High Blood Pressure, U.S. Department of Health and Human Services, National Institutes of Health, National Heart, Lung, and Blood Institute, Rockville, MD, May, 2003.
91. National Cholesterol Education Program, Third Report of the National Cholesterol Education Program (NCEP) Expert Panel on Detection, Evaluation, and Treatment of High Blood Cholesterol in Adults (Adult Treatment Panel III), U.S. Department of Health and Human Services, National Institutes of Health, National Heart, Lung, and Blood Institute, Rockville, MD, September, 2002.
92. National Research Council Food and Nutrition Board, *Toward Healthful Diets,* The National Research Council, National Academy of Science, Washington, DC, 1980.
93. United States Department of Agriculture and United States Department of Health and Human Services, *Nutrition and Your Health: Dietary Guidelines for Americans,* 3rd ed., Home and Garden Bulletin, Number 232, United States Printing Office, Washington, DC, 1990.
94. United States Department of Agriculture, Report of the Dietary Guidelines Advisory Committee on the Dietary Guidelines for Americans, National Technical Information Service, 1995.
95. United States Department of Agriculture and the United States Department of Health and Human Services, *Nutrition and Your Health: The Food Guide Pyramid,* 3rd ed., Home and Garden Bulletin, Number 252, United States Government Printing Office, Washington, DC, 1990.
96. United States Department of Agriculture, Center for Nutrition Policy and Promotion, Dietary Guidelines for Americans, United States Government Printing Office, Washington, DC, 2005.
97. Wardlaw, G.M., *Contemporary Nutrition,* 6th ed., McGraw-Hill Higher Education, New York, 2006.
98. Wardlaw, G.M. and M.W. Kessel, *Perspectives in Nutrition,* 5th ed., McGraw-Hill, New York, 2002.
99. Whitney, E.N., C.B. Cataldo, and S.R. Rolfes, *Understanding Normal and Clinical Nutrition,* 7th ed., Wadsworth/Thomson Learning, Stamford, CT, 2006.
100. Wilson, P.W.F., Homocysteine and coronary heart disease: how great is the hazard? *Journal of the American Medical Association,* 288, 2042–2043, 2002.
101. Wyatt, H.R. et al., A Colorado statewide survey of walking and its relation to excessive weight, *Medicine and Science in Sport and Exercise,* 37, 724–730,2005.
102. Yusuf, S. et al., Obesity and the risk of myocardial infarction in 27,000 participants from 6 countries: a case-control study, *Lancet,* 366, 9497, 2005.
103. Zubrod, G. and J.R. Holman, Novel biochemical markers of cardiovascular risk: a primary care primer, *Consultant,* 44, 1509–1513, October, 2004.

10 Obesity and Heart Disease

INTRODUCTION

In the United States heart disease ranks as the leading cause of death.[47] In this regard, obesity has become a major risk factor.[49] The relative risk of obesity to heart disease has been substantially investigated. Over the years, height/weight tables, ratios, and indices have been developed to measure the range of normal to abnormal weight levels. Research has been focused on the relationship of excess weight to heart disease. This relationship has been reported to be curvilinear in nature and gradated within the parameters of increasing body mass index height–weight levels to rising heart disease rates.[11,69] With more than 66 and 32% of American men and women 20 years and older found to be overweight and obese, respectively, in 2003–2004, the significance of excess weight has become a prevalent and rising health problem relative to the morbidity and mortality of heart disease (Figure 10.1).[39,46,48,51,62,64,67,70,71,72]

OBESITY TYPES

Four obesity phenotypes have been designated by Bouchard (Figure 10.2).[7,9,53] Type One obesity is characterized by an overall excess bodily mass or fat. Type Two is described as an android adiposity with excess fat located in the truncal and abdominal body regions. Type Three pertains to the centralized abdominal fat located in the visceral area of the body. The last, Type Four is found in the gluteal and thigh regions of the body and is characterized as gynoid-related fat patterning. These obesity types are measured, assessed, and classified through the utilization of height-weight tables, height-weight ratios, and waist-hip circumference ratios. Type One obesity reflects overall body fat patterning while Types Two, Three, and Four are descriptive of regional fat depositions.

CAUSES OF OBESITY

The causes of obesity are genetically and environmentally interrelated. Genetically, excess weight has been related to the inheritance of obesity genes, body build, and regional body fat distribution.[8,16,70] Studies have shown that obesity may be genetically predisposed.[16] Gene inheritance in this regard may involve a combination of genes that may be the coding determinant for thinness to fatness relative to body weight.

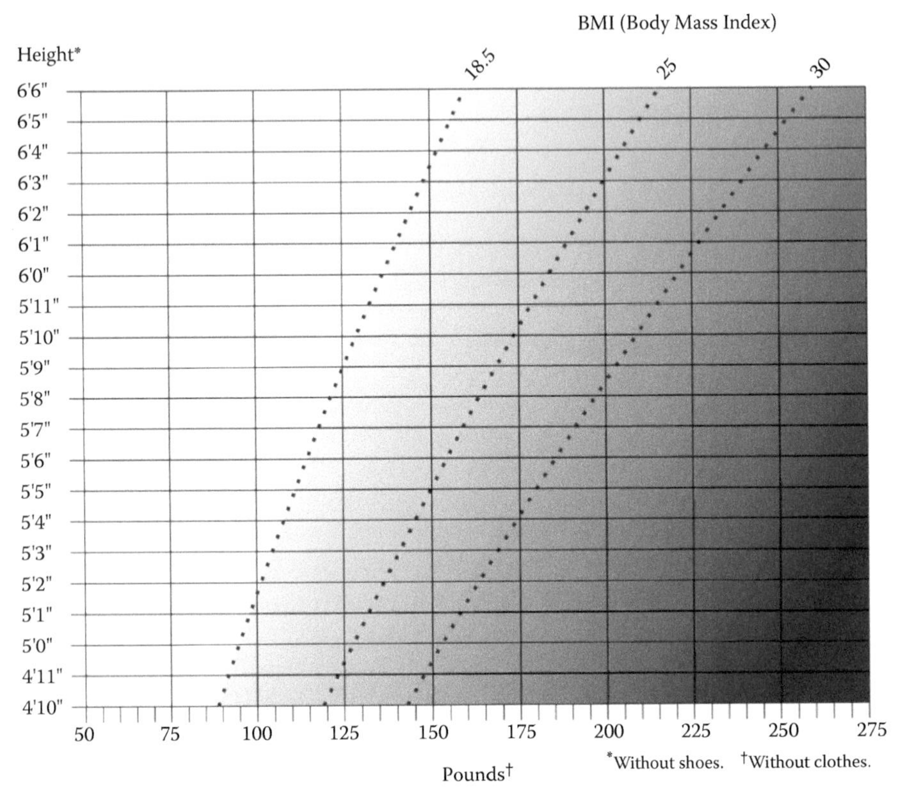

BMI measures weight in relation to height. The BMI ranges shown above are for adults. They are not exact ranges of healthy and unhealthy weights. However, they show that health risk increases at higher levels of overweight and obesity. Even within the healthy BMI range, weight gains can carry health risks for adults.

Directions: Find your weight on the bottom of the graph. Go straight up from that point until you come to the line that matches your height. Then look to find your weight group.

Healthy Weight BMI from 18.5 up to 25 refers to healthy weight.

Overweight BMI from 25 up to 30 refers to overweight.

Obese BMI 30 or higher refers to obesity. Obese persons are also overweight.

Source: Report of the Dietary Guidelines Advisory Committee on the Dietary Guidelines for Americans, 2000, page 3.

FIGURE 10.1 Body mass index weight chart. (From United States Department of Agriculture, Report of the Dietary Guidelines Advisory Committee on the Dietary Guidelines for Americans, 2000, United States Department of Agriculture, 2000.)

Type 1 Obesity:	Excess Body Mass or Percent Fat
Type 2 Obesity:	Excess Subcutaneous Truncal-Abdominal Fat (Android)
Type 3 Obesity:	Excess Abdominal Visceral Fat
Type 4 Obesity:	Excess Gluteo-Femoral Fat (Gynoid)

FIGURE 10.2 The types of obesity phenotypes in a health perspective. (Source: General Mills Inc., *Contemporary Nutrition,* 15, 10, 1990. Reprinted with permission.)

Twin studies have corroborated this genetic predisposition. When reared apart, twins have reportedly demonstrated similar weight gain patterns within similar weight range levels.[65,66,67] Similarly, parents that are overweight and obese may also pass on these genetic traits to their children. Body build has been reported to be genetically influenced.[7,8,9] Endomorphic and mesomorphic children that are overweight and muscular would be predisposed to greater weight gain patterns than would their ectomorphic sibling counterparts.[67] Mesomorphy has been found to have a higher heritability factor than endomorphy and ectomorphy.[7] In addition, regional body fat distribution may also be predisposed genetically relative to android and gynoid-type fat depositions.[7,70]

Earlier studies on genetic regulation of body weight were related to fat cell development and set point metabolism. In reference to fat cell development, the number and size of these cells acquired prior to birth, during infancy, and in adolescence resulted in a weight gain pattern that exceeded normal levels during growth.[54,68,70] While the size of these fat cells were regulated to some extent through diet and exercise, the existing number remained and did not change.[6,71] Increasing obesity in this regard was characterized by fat cell size increase to set limits, and the development of new fat cells when these size limits were reached.[70] The enzymatic activity of lipoprotein lipase governed the rate of storage in these fat cells.[66] Obesity and lipoprotein lipase activity were interrelated. The greater the weight, the greater the lipoprotein lipase fat storage activity. Two types of obesity fat cells were categorized. Hyperplastic obesity was designated by a greater than average number of fat cells, while hypertrophic obesity was denoted by fat cells that were larger than normal in size.[70] The genetic predisposition to set point range weight regulation was related to metabolic rate. This process was monitored by hypothalamic homeostatic stability activity in the governance of appetite and eventual weight range controls.[66] When weight was lost and lower set point limits were reached, metabolic rate was slowed in order to maintain lower weight levels, whereas when weight was gained and higher set point limits were attained, metabolic rate was accelerated in order to stay within higher weight range levels.

Environmentally, energy balance and physical inactivity have contributed to weight gaining processes.[14,15,65] The energy balance of caloric intake and caloric utilization are interrelated and can regulate weight gain, weight maintenance, and weight loss within given limits. In reference to physical activity, studies have demonstrated an evidential relationship between exercise, weight control, and subsequent related mortality disease risks (Table 10.1 and Figure 10.3).[46,48] The research has

TABLE 10.1
Association of Physical Activity and Cardiac Mortality

	Energy Expenditure (Kcal/Week):				
Kind of Activity	<150	150-399	400-749	750-1,499	≥1,500
Vigorous activity					
No. of CHD deaths	180	151	52	41	41
RR	1.00	0.94	0.77	0.89	0.68
95% confidence interval	referent	0.76-1.17	0.56-1.06	0.63-1.26	0.48-0.96
Nonvigorous activity					
No. of CHD deaths	56	89	95	110	115
RR	1.00	1.15	1.10	1.12	0.89
95% confidence interval	referent	0.82-1.61	0.79-1.53	0.81-1.54	0.64-1.23

Source: From United States Department of Health and Human Services, *Physical Activity and Health: A Report of the Surgeon General,* United States Department of Health and Human Services, Centers for Disease Control and Prevention, 1996. With permission.

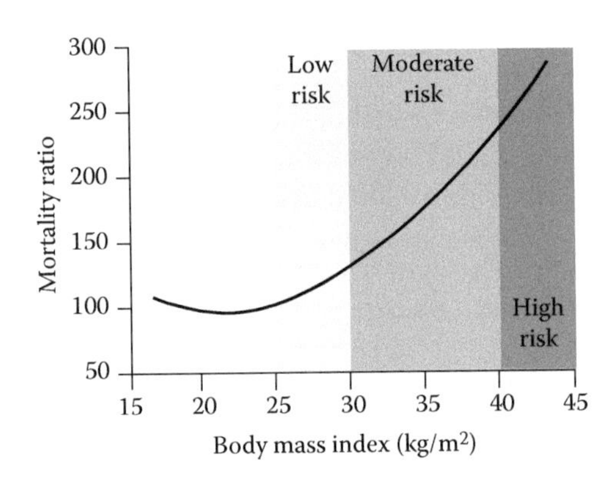

FIGURE 10.3 Body mass index levels and mortality risks. (From Robergs, R.A. and S.A. Roberts, *Exercise Physiology: Exercise, Performance, and Clinical Applications,* Mosby, Philadelphia, 1997. With permission from Elsevier.)

been centered on dose–response studies relative to the amount and level of exercise that would promote an effect on both excess body weight and overall health. According to Di Pietro,[15] studies showed that physical activity promoted fat loss and conserved lean body weight, that the weight loss was related to the duration and intensity of the exercise, and that the weight loss was slow but effective in the control of weight.

HEIGHT-WEIGHT TABLES

The modern concept of desirable body weight originated with the Medico-Actuarial Mortality Investigations published by life insurance companies in 1912.[1] The purpose of these investigations was to establish standard height-weight tables that reflected weight as a percentage of designated norms for those of the same height, age, and sex. These tables delineated desirable to undesirable weight ranges relative to health as well as to disease, morbidity, and mortality rates. In the early twentieth century, higher premiums were mandated for those who were thin, since linearity of body build was highly related to tuberculosis. This practice changed after the insurance investigations were conducted. It was found that those heaviest in weight for given height and age levels had greater mortality risk than those who were lighter in weight.

Further advances in this area were made through the 1959 Build and Blood Pressure Study[10] and the 1979 Build Study.[50] In the 1959 study,[10] frame sizes were arbitrarily established in order to offset the problem of the large diversity in weight levels. Weight ranges were initiated for each of the frame sizes. Desirable weights for men were set at 5 feet in height and 110 pounds in weight and for women at 5 ft. and 100 pounds. Each inch beyond 5 feet in height carried a 5-pound addition in weight. Subsequent evaluations of the weight ranges and ideal weights were later found to be too low.[69] Based on the 1979 study,[50] the 1983 Metropolitan Height and Weight table reflected 10- to 15-pound increases in the revised weight levels.[45,50] The average relative weight for Americans was also increased and set at 1.20 or 20% above the ideal weight standard. Frame size approximations similar to those of the 1959 study were utilized.[43] Anthropometric determinations were later adopted based on the data results of the NHANES Studies I and II.[43] The results of the 1979 study showed mortality risks to be greatest for those in the extreme overweight and underweight categories.[47]

The controversial nature of the results, however, prompted critical appraisals of the 1979 study. Knapp[38] reported that the 1979 results were controversial relative to the establishment of desirable weight criteria, the quality of the obtained data, and the lack of a representative sample. Lee and Nieman[43] designated that there were limitations in the control of the variables, the determination of the frame sizes, and the lack of body composition data. Similarly, Russell et al.[55] stated that the study reflected only given populations and present average values for those populations, and would not be applicable to different time frames of reference. However, the frame size categories and weight range levels have been accepted and utilized as practical and approximate references in the screening of underweight to overweight persons relative to possible clinical and disease risk factors.[67]

HEIGHT-WEIGHT RATIOS

Height-weight ratio formulations have also been used as measures of weight, obesity, and bodily frame size. While these ratios provided data similar to those expressed by height-weight tables, they were also indicative of the trend toward the use of continuous quantitative measures of relative weight that facilitated individual comparisons to the general population. Two of the more frequently used ratios have been those developed by Livi[44] and Quetelet.[35] Livi[44] introduced an index that incorporated the cube root of weight divided by height in order to describe what he termed the indice ponderale (ponderal index) or bodily frame size. The Quetelet index, as reported by Keys et al.,[35] combined a weight divided by height squared ratio to

TABLE 10.2
Body Mass Index Table

BMI	19	20	21	22	23	24	25	26	27	28	29	30	31	32	33	34	35
Height (inches)								Body Weight (pounds)									
58	91	96	100	105	110	115	119	124	129	134	138	143	148	153	158	162	167
59	94	99	104	109	114	119	124	128	133	138	143	148	153	158	163	168	173
60	97	102	107	112	118	123	128	133	138	143	148	153	158	163	168	174	179
61	100	106	111	116	122	127	132	137	143	148	153	158	164	169	174	180	185
62	104	109	115	120	126	131	136	142	147	153	158	164	169	175	180	186	191
63	107	113	118	124	130	135	141	146	152	158	163	169	175	180	186	191	197
64	110	116	122	128	134	140	145	151	157	163	169	174	180	186	192	197	204
65	114	120	126	132	138	144	150	156	162	168	174	180	186	192	198	204	210
66	118	124	130	136	142	148	155	161	167	173	179	186	192	198	204	210	216
67	121	127	134	140	146	153	159	166	172	178	185	191	198	204	211	217	223
68	125	131	138	144	151	158	164	171	177	184	190	197	203	210	216	223	230
69	128	135	142	149	155	162	169	176	182	189	196	203	209	216	223	230	236
70	132	139	146	153	160	167	174	181	188	195	202	209	216	222	229	236	243
71	136	143	150	157	165	172	179	186	193	200	208	215	222	229	236	243	250
72	140	147	154	162	169	177	184	191	199	206	213	221	228	235	242	250	258
73	144	151	159	166	174	182	189	197	204	212	219	227	235	242	250	257	265
74	148	155	163	171	179	186	194	202	210	218	225	233	241	249	256	264	272
75	152	160	168	176	184	192	200	208	216	224	232	240	248	256	264	272	279
76	156	164	172	180	189	197	205	213	221	230	238	246	254	263	271	279	287

Source: From National Institutes of Health, National Heart, Lung and Blood Institute, *The Practical Guide: Identification, Evaluation, and Treatment of Overweight and Obesity in Adults,* National Institutes of Health, National Heart, Lung, and Blood Institute, NIH Publication No. 00–4084, October, 2000.

designate what was termed a body mass index. Both of these indices have been extensively used by researchers and have become known as standard measures for frame size and body mass.[29,36,50,57] Criteria for the development of indices of this type were also advanced. Benn[2] reported that height-weight ratios should be highly related to other measures of relative fatness and should demonstrate a noncorrelation with height. Height was to be utilized as a corrective figure, since weight was not constant with an increase in height relative to form and shape.

The body mass index[36,42,48] was found to be highly related to weight and body skinfold fatness, and significantly independent of height. The ponderal index was found to be negatively correlated with weight and dependent upon height.[36] The body mass index translated weight levels into underweight, desirable and overweight ranges for both men and women. Desirable indices were set at 22.7 for men and at 22.4 for women.[24] These index weight ranges were recently changed in a report published by the National Institutes of Health on overweight and obesity.[49] Set ranges between 18.5 and 24.9 reflected desirable weight, 25 to 29.9 overweight, and 30 and greater obesity (Table 10.2, Table 10.3, and Table 10.4).[11] Indices set between 20 and 25 have been generally shown to be related to greater longevity than those set above this range standard.[24] Measures comparative to the body mass index and the ponderal index have also been developed and investigated. Khosla and Lowe[36] devised an index based on weight divided by height cubed (derived from Sheldon's height-divided-by-the-cube-root-of-weight ratio) while Benn[3] formulated a ratio based on weight divided by height with a power derivative (power equals a population-specific-source). Lee et al.[42] reported that the index derived by Khosla and

TABLE 10.3
Body Mass Index Table

BMI	36	37	38	39	40	41	42	43	44	45	46	47	48	49	50	51	52	53	54
58	172	177	181	186	191	196	201	205	210	215	220	224	229	234	239	244	248	253	258
59	178	183	188	193	198	203	208	212	217	222	227	232	237	242	247	252	257	262	267
60	184	189	194	199	204	209	215	220	225	230	235	240	245	250	255	261	266	271	276
61	190	195	201	206	211	217	222	227	232	238	243	248	254	259	264	269	275	280	285
62	196	202	207	213	218	224	229	235	240	246	251	256	262	267	273	278	284	289	295
63	203	208	214	220	225	231	237	242	248	254	259	265	270	278	282	287	293	299	304
64	209	215	221	227	232	238	244	250	256	262	267	273	279	285	291	296	302	308	314
65	216	222	228	234	240	246	252	258	264	270	276	282	288	294	300	306	312	318	324
66	223	229	235	241	247	253	260	266	272	278	284	291	297	303	309	315	322	328	334
67	230	236	242	249	255	261	268	274	280	287	293	299	306	312	319	325	331	338	344
68	236	243	249	256	262	269	276	282	289	295	302	308	315	322	328	335	341	348	354
69	243	250	257	263	270	277	284	291	297	304	311	318	324	331	338	345	351	358	365
70	250	257	264	271	278	285	292	299	306	313	320	327	334	341	348	355	362	369	376
71	257	265	272	279	286	293	301	308	315	322	329	338	343	351	358	365	372	379	386
72	265	272	279	287	294	302	309	316	324	331	338	346	353	361	368	375	383	390	397
73	272	280	288	295	302	310	318	325	333	340	348	355	363	371	378	386	393	401	408
74	280	287	295	303	311	319	326	334	342	350	358	365	373	381	389	396	404	412	420
75	287	295	303	311	319	327	335	343	351	359	367	375	383	391	399	407	415	423	431
76	295	304	312	320	328	336	344	353	361	369	377	385	394	402	410	418	426	435	443

Source: From National Institutes of Health, National Heart, Lung and Blood Institute, *The Practical Guide: Identification, Evaluation, and Treatment of Overweight and Obesity in Adults,* National Institutes of Health, National Heart, Lung, and Blood Institute, NIH Publication No. 00-4084, October, 2000.

TABLE 10.4

Body Mass Index

Weight in Kilograms Divided by Height in Meters Squared

Obesity Greater Than 30 ____________________

Overweight 25 – 29.9 ____________________

Desirable Weight 18.5 – 24.9 ____________________

Underweight Less than 18.5 ____________________

Source: Adapted from National Institutes of Health, National Heart, Lung and Blood Institute, *The Practical Guide: Identification, Evaluation, and Treatment of Overweight and Obesity in Adults,* National Institutes of Health, National Heart, Lung, and Blood Institute, NIH Publication No. 00-4084, October, 2000.

Lowe[36] was moderately related to weight but influenced by height, whereas the Benn index was highly correlated to weight and independent of height.

FRAME SIZE

In reference to frame size, classifications are generally derivatives of height/breadth measurement formulations. The resulting ratios are utilized in the form of indices which denote the nature and range of the types. Three types have been developed within variational parameters and can be identified as small, medium, and large. The criteria for frame size classification has been limited to a measure of the basic build of the body or the skeletal and fat-free mass that would be independent of height and not related to fat weight.[3,21,33] These criteria however, may not be acceptable, since lean body and fat body weight may be interdependent.[2,17] Recent measures have been developed by Katch and Freedson,[33] Garn et al.,[22] and Frisancho and Flegel.[21] Katch and Freedson[33] used what they termed a mathematical model based on the correlation of height with the sum of the biacromial and bitrochanteric diameter landmark measures. Small, medium, and large body sizes were computed relative to percentile ranking of body weight, fat percentage, and lean body weight. Bony chest breadth was used by Garn et al.[22] as their criterion measure for frame size. Small, medium and large chest categories were formed to measure fat-free body mass and relative fatness. Frisancho and Flegel[21] utilized sex, race, and age-specific percentiles of elbow breadth to classify subjects into frame size categories of small, medium, and large. Frisancho,[20] in a later study, also categorized frame size through the use of biacromial and bitrochanteric breadth measurements.

Height-weight tables and ratios have been used extensively in the study of the relationships of body build to blood lipids, atherosclerosis, and heart disease. Standard measures of this type have provided continuous quantitative scales, facilitated group comparisons, and have enabled investigators to study large numbers of subjects.

OBESITY AND HEART DISEASE

Early studies relating body build to heart disease utilized somatotype and anthropometric index rating measures of assessment. Males with mesomorphic muscularity and endomorphic fatness were found to be more predisposed to higher cholesterol levels and atherosclerosis than those with ectomorphic thinness.[13,18,25,28,59,61] Similarly, the body size indices of males exhibiting shortness in height, sturdiness in build, and heaviness in weight were also reported to be highly related to the development of atherosclerosis and heart disease.[14,15,34,32,41]

Recent studies in this area have been directed toward the use of body mass indices and regional body fat localization rating measures to denote the coronary disease relationship.[64] Cardiovascular disease risk has been found to be related to high cholesterol, low-density lipoprotein levels, and to decreased levels of high-density lipoproteins.[27] Excess weight in both men and women has been reportedly shown to be one of the predominant factors in this relationship of increased coronary disease risk.[23,30,40,47,46,49] The high body mass indices of the men and women in these studies showed a positive relationship to low-density and a negative relationship to high-density lipoprotein cholesterol. High body mass indices were also found to be significantly related to heart failure.[35]

In reference to regional body fat localization, studies have generally shown adiposity in men (android) to be centered mainly in the abdomen, whereas fat in women (gynoid) was located in the abdominal, gluteal, and thigh regions of the body.[16,19,39,49,52,60] Abdominal obesity and upper body fat distribution patterns in both men and women can predispose them to higher cholesterol and triglyceride levels and to a greater risk of heart disease.[4,5,6,11,34,37,38] Studies in this regard have deonstrated this relationship and have set waist–gluteal circumference ratio measurements at 0.85 for women and 0.95 for men (Table 10.5 and Table 10.6).[4,5,12,62]

In addition to the waist-hip ratio relationship to heart disease, abdominal fat as measured by waist circumference has also been advanced as an independent risk factor (Table 10.7).[48,56,64] Excess fat in the abdominal region that is proportionally predominant to overall fat would be indicative of an increased obesity risk to heart disease.[48] Risk relationship figures have been set at waist circumference measures of greater than 40 inches for men and 35 inches for women relative to body mass indices of 25 to 34.9.[48] Similarly, a recent study by Smith and associates found an abdominal diameter index to be related to an increased heart disease risk.[58]

SUMMARY

The conclusions drawn from the studies cited indicate that:

1. Approximately 33% of American men and women between the ages of 20 and 74 have been categorized as excessively weighted during the period of 1988–1991.
2. This excessiveness in weight has become a prevalent and rising health problem relative to the morbidity and mortality of heart disease.
3. Four obesity types have been determined. Type One obesity reflects overall body fat patterning. Types Two, Three, and Four are descriptive of regional fat depositions.
4. The causes of obesity are genetically and environmentally interrelated
5. Genetically, excess weight has been related to the inheritance of obesity genes, body build, regional body fat distribution, fat cell development, and metabolic set point weight regulation.
6. Environmentally, energy balance and physical inactivity can contribute to weight gaining processes.
7. Height-weight tables and height-weight ratios may be utilized in the assessment of desirable and undesirable weight levels and as indicators of health risks.
8. Endomorphy and mesomorphy are positively related to high cholesterol levels.

TABLE 10.5
Waist/Hip Ratio

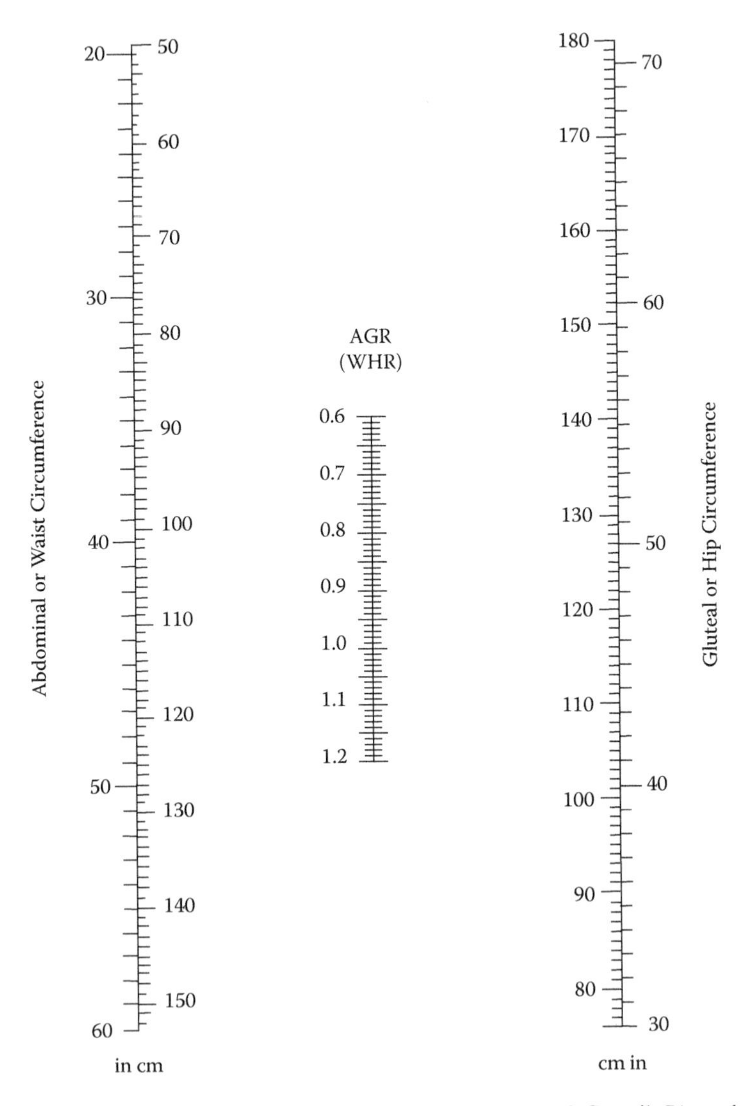

Source: From Committee on Diet and Health, National Research Council, *Diet and Health: Implications for Reducing Chronic Disease Risk,* The National Academy of Sciences, The National Academies Press, Washington, DC, 1989. With permission.

TABLE 10.6
Waist/Hip Ratio

Waist Circumference
(Inches)

———

Hip Circumference
(Inches)

———

Waist / Hip Ratio

———

Men -	**<.85 Desirable**
Women -	**<.95 Desirable**

Source: Adapted from National Institutes of Health, National Heart, Lung and Blood Institute, *The Practical Guide: Identification, Evaluation, and Treatment of Overweight and Obesity in Adults,* National Institutes of Health, National Heart, Lung, and Blood Institute, NIH Publication No.00-4084, October, 2000.

TABLE 10.7
Waist Circumference (Inches)

Men	-	**<40 Desirable**
Women	-	**<35 Desirable**

Source: Adapted from National Institutes of Health, National Heart, Lung and Blood Institute, *The Practical Guide: Identification, Evaluation, and Treatment of Overweight and Obesity in Adults,* National Institutes of Health, National Heart, Lung, and Blood Institute, NIH Publication No.00-4084, October, 2000.

9. The body size characteristics of shortness in height, sturdiness in body build, and heaviness in weight are related to high cholesterol levels, the development of atherosclerosis, and cardiovascular disease in both men and women.
10. In reference to cholesterol fractionation findings, (high-density and low-density lipoproteins), slimness in body build is favorably associated with increasing levels of high-density lipoprotein cholesterol, and obesity with decreasing levels of the component in both men and women.
11. Excessive upper body fat in the abdominal region is related to high triglyceride levels and ischemic heart disease.

GLOSSARY

Body mass index (quetelet index) Body weight in kilograms divided by height in meters squared

Frame size The basic build or the skeletal and lean mass of the body determined by the proportional relationship of height to one or more breadth measures

Hyperplastic obesity Characterized by fat cells that are greater in size than normal

Hypertrophic obesity Characterized by greater than an average number of fat cells

Lipoprotein lipase activity An enzymatic process that governs the bodily storage of fat in cells

Obesity phenotypes Type One obesity is characterized by an overall excess bodily mass or fat.

Ponderal index (Livi index) Height divided by the cube root of weight

Type Two is described as an android adiposity with excess fat located in the truncal and abdominal body regions.

Type Three pertains to the centralized abdominal fat located in the visceral area of the body.

Type Four is found in the gluteal and thigh regions of the body and is characterized as gynoid-related fat patterning.

Waist/hip ratio The circumference of the abdomen divided by the circumference of the hips or gluteal region of the body

REFERENCES

1. Association of Life Insurance Medical Directors, *Medico-Actuarial Mortality Investigations,* Vol. 1, Associated Life Insurance Medical Directors and Actuaries Society of America, Chicago, 1912.
2. Battinelli, T. Frame size: a type and subtype approach, *Journal of Obesity and Weight Regulation,* 8, 67–76, 1989.
3. Benn, R.T., Some mathematical properties of weight-for-height indices used as measures of adiposity, *British Journal of Preventive Social Medicine,* 25, 42–50, 1971.

4. Bjorntorp, P., Hazards in subgroups of human obesity, *European Journal of Clinical Investigation,* 14, 239–241, 1984.
5. Bjorntorp, P., Regional patterns of fat distribution, *Annals of Internal Medicine,* 103, 994–995, 1985.
6. Bjorntorp, P., U. Smith, and P. Lonsroth, Health implications of regional obesity, *Acta Medica Scandinavica Symposium,* Series No. 4, Almqvist and Wiksese Institutional, Stockholm, 1998.
7. Bouchard, C., Genetic influences of body composition and regional fat distribution, *Contemporary Nutrition,* 15, 1–2, 1990.
8. Bouchard, C., Heredity and the path to overweight and obesity, *Medicine and Science in Sports and Exercise,* 25, 285–291, 1991.
9. Bouchard, C., Long-term programming of body size, *Nutrition Reviews,* 54, S8–S14, February, 1996.
10. Association of Life Insurance Medical Directors and the Society of Actuaries, *Build and Blood Pressure Study,* Vols. 1 and 2, Association of Life Insurance Medical Directors and the Society of Actuaries, Chicago, 1959.
11. Burton, B.T. and W.R. Foster, Health implications of obesity: an NIH Consensus Development Conference: perspectives in practice, *American Dietetic Association,* 85, 1117–1121, 1985.
12. Bray, G.A., Pathophysiology of obesity, *American Journal of Clinical Nutrition,* 55, 488S-494S, 1992.
13. Carter, J.E.L. and B.H. Heath, *Somatotyping-Development and Applications,* Cambridge University Press, Cambridge, 1990.
14. Clark, T.D. and J.R. Holman, Obesity: is there effective treatment, *Consultant,* 46, 301–309, March, 2006.
15. Di Pietro, L., Physical activity in the prevention of obesity: current evidence and research issues, *Medicine and Science in Sport and Exercise,* 31, S542-S546, 1999.
16. Fackelmann, K.A., Family ties point to recessive obesity gene, *Science News,* 136, 327, November 18, 1989.
17. Forbes, G.G. and S.L. Welle, Lean body mass in obesity, *International Journal of Obesity,* 7, 99–107, 1983.
18. Forssman, O. and B. Lindegard, The post-coronary patient; a multidisciplinary investigation of middle-aged Swedish males, *Journal of Psychosomatic Research,* 3, 89–169, 1958.
19. Freedman, D.S. et al., Body fat distribution and male/female differences in lipids and lipoproteins, *Circulation,* 81, 1498–1505, May, 1990.
20. Frisancho, A.R., *Anthropometric Standards for the Assessment of Growth and Nutritional Status,* University of Michigan Press, Ann Arbor, MI, 1990.
21. Frisancho, A.R. and P.N. Flegel, Elbow breadth as a measure of frame size for U.S. males and females, *American Journal of Clinical Nutrition,* 37, 311–314, 1983.
22. Garn, S.M. et al., The bony chest breadth as a frame size standard in nutritional assessment, *American Journal of Clinical Nutrition,* 37, 315–318, 1983.
23. Garrison, R.J. et al., Obesity and lipoprotein cholesterol in the Framingham Offspring Study, *Metabolism,* 29, 1053–1060, 1980.
24. Garrow, J.S., Indices of adiposity, *Nutrition Abstracts and Reviews,* 53, 697–708, 1983.
25. Gertler, M.M., S.M. Garn, and H.B. Sprague, Cholesterol, cholesterol esters and phospholipids in health and in coronary artery disease morphology and serum lipids, *Circulation,* 2, 380–381, 1950.

26. Grosvenor, M.B. and L.A. Smolin, *Nutrition: Everyday Choices,* John Wiley and Sons Incorporated, New York, 2006.
27. Grundy, S.M., Cholesterol and coronary heart disease: future directions, *Journal of the American Medical Association,* 264, 3053–3059, December 19, 1990.
28. Harrison, G.A. et al., *Human Biology: An Introduction to Human Evolution, Growth, and Adaptability,* 3rd ed., Oxford University Press, Oxford, 1990.
29. Heath, B.M. and J.E.L. Carter, A modified somatotype method, *American Journal of Physical Anthropology,* 27, 57–74, 1967.
30. Hoffmans, M.D., D. Kromhout, and C.D. Coulander, Body mass index at the age of 18 and its effects on 32-year-mortality from coronary heart disease and cancer, a nested case-control study among the entire 1932 Dutch male birth cohort, *Journal of Clinical Epidemiology,* 42, 513–520, 1989.
31. Hrubic, Z. and W.J. Zukel, Epidemiology of coronary heart disease among young army males of World War II. *American Heart Journal,* 87, 722–730, 1974.
32. Kannel, W.B., C. Pearson, and P.M. McNamara, Obesity as a force of morbidity. In *Adolescent Nutrition and Growth,* Heath, P., Ed., Appleton-Century-Crofts, New York, 1969.
33. Katch, V.L. and P.S. Freedson, Body size and shape: derivation of the "hat" frame size model, *American Journal of Clinical Nutrition,* 36, 669–675, 1982.
34. Kaye, S.A. et al., The association of body fat distribution with life-style and reproductive factors in a population study of postmenopausal women, *International Journal of Obesity,* 14, 583–591, 1990.
35. Kenchaiah, S. et al., Obesity and the risk of heart failure, *New England Journal of Medicine,* 347(5), 305–313, August 1, 2002.
36. Khosla, T. and C.R. Lowe, Indices of obesity derived from body weight and height, *British Journal of Preventive Social Medicine,* 21, 122–128, 1967.
37. Kissebah, A.H. et al., Relation of body fat distribution to metabolic complications of obesity, *Journal of Clinical Endocrinology and Metabolism,* 54, 254–260, 1982.
38. Knapp, T.R., A methodological critique of the ideal weight concept, *Journal of the American Medical Association,* 250, 506–510, 1983.
39. Kuczmarski, R.J. et al., Increasing prevalence of overweight among U.S. adults: the National Health and Nutrition Examination Surveys, 1960–1991, *Journal of the American Medical Association,* 272, 205–211, July 20, 1994.
40. Larsson, B. et al., Abdominal adipose tissue distribution, obesity, and risk of cardiovascular disease and death: 13 year follow up of participants in the study of men born in 1913, *British Medical Journal,* 288, 1401–1404, May 12, 1984.
41. Lee, I.M. et al., Body weight and mortality: a 27-year follow-up of middle-aged men, *Journal of American Medical Association,* 270, 2823–2828, December 15, 1993.
42. Lee, J., L.N. Kolonel, and M.W. Hinds, Relative merits of the weight-corrected-for-height indices, *American Journal of Clinical Nutrition,* 34, 2521–2529, 1981.
43. Lee, R.D. and D.C. Nieman, *Nutritional Assessment,* Brown and Benchmark, Madison, WI, 1993.
44. Livi, R.L., Indice Ponderale O Rapporto Tra La Statura E il Peso, *Atti Societa Romana Antropologia,* 5, 125–153, 1897.
45. Manson, J.E. and S.S. Bassuk, Obesity in the United States: a fresh look at its high toll, *Journal of the American Medical Association,* 289, 229–230, 2003.
46. McInnis, K.J., B.A. Franklin, and J.M. Rippe, Counseling for physical activity in overweight and obese patients, *American Family Physician,* 67, 1249–1256, 2003.
47. Metropolitan Life Insurance Company, *Metropolitan Height and Weight Tables,* New York, Metropolitan Life Insurance Company, 1983.

48. National Institutes of Health, National Institutes of Health Consensus Development Conference Statement, Health implications of obesity, *Annals of Internal Medicine,* 103, 1073–1077, 1985.
49. National Institutes of Health, National Heart, Lung and Blood Institute, The Practical Guide: Identification, Evaluation, and Treatment of Overweight and Obesity in Adults, National Heart, Lung and Blood Institute, NIH Publication No. 00–4084, October, 2000.
50. Society of Actuaries and Association of Life Insurance Medical Directors of America, *1979 Build Study,* Society of Actuaries and Association of Life Insurance, Chicago, 1980.
51. Ogden, C.L. et al., Prevalence of overweight and obesity in the United States, 1999–2004, *Journal of the American Medical Association,* 295(13), 1549–1555, April 5, 2006.
52. President's Council on Physical Fitness and Sport, Exercise obesity, and weight control, *Physical Activity and Fitness Research Digest,* Washington, DC, 1994.
53. President's Council on Physical Fitness and Sport, Heredity and health-related fitness, *Physical Activity and Fitness Research Digest,* Washington, DC, 1993.
54. Robergs, R.A. and S.J. Keteyian, *Fundamentals of Exercise Physiology for Fitness, Performance, and Health,* 2nd ed., McGraw-Hill Higher Education, New York, 2003.
55. Russell, R.M., R.B. McGandy, and D. Jellife, Reference weights: practical considerations, *American Journal of Medicine,* 76, 767–769, 1985.
56. Sharma, A.M., The obese patient with diabetes mellitus: from research targets to treatment options, *American Journal of Medicine,* 119(5A), 17S–23S, 2006.
57. Sheldon, W.H., S.S. Stevens, and W.B. Tucker, *The Varieties of Human Physique,* Harper and Brothers, New York, 1940.
58. Smith, D.A., Abdominal diameter index, clinical capsules, *Internal Medicine News,* 38, 33, August 1, 2003.
59. Spain, D.M., V.A. Bradess, and J.J. Greenblatt, Post-mortem studies on coronary atherosclerosis, serum beta lipoprotein, and somatotypes, *American Journal of Medical Science,* 229, 294–301, 1955.
60. Tanasescu, M. et al., Exercise type and intensity in relation to coronary heart disease in men, *Journal of the American Medical Association,* 288, 1994–2000, 2002.
61. Tanner, J.M., Relationship between serum cholesterol and physique in healthy young men, *Journal of Physiology,* 115, 371–390, 1951.
62. The Institute of Food Technologists' Expert Panel on Food Safety and Nutrition, Human obesity, *Contemporary Nutrition,* 16, 1–4, 1993.
63. Thompson, J. and M. Manore, *Nutrition: An Applied Approach,* Pearson Education, San Francisco, 2005.
64. United States Department of Agriculture, *Report of the Dietary Guidelines Advisory Committee on the Dietary Guidelines for Americans,* National Technical Information Services, 1995.
65. Volek, J.S., J.L. VanHeest, and C.E. Forsythe, Diet and exercise for weight loss: a review of the current issues, *Sports Medicine,* 36, 1–9, 2005.
66. Wardlaw, G.M. and M. Kessel, *Perspectives in Nutrition,* 5th ed., McGraw-Hill, New York, 2002.
67. Wardlaw, G.M., *Contemporary Nutrition,* 6th ed. McGraw-Hill, New York, 2006.
68. Weinstein, A.R. and H.D. Sesso, Joint effects of physical activity and body weight on diabetes and cardiovascular disease, *Exercise and Sport Sciences Reviews,* 34, 10–15, 2006.
69. Whitney, E.N. and S.R. Rolfs, *Understanding Nutrition,* 10th ed., Thomson/Wadsworth, Belmont, CA, 2005.

70. Williams, M.H., *Nutrition for Health, Fitness, and Sport,* 7th ed., McGraw-Hill Higher Education, New York, 2005.
71. Wilmore, J.H. and D.L. Costill, *Physiology of Sport and Exercise,* 3rd ed., Human Kinetics, Champaign, IL, 2004.
72. Yanovski, S.Z., K. Donato, and L. Garisheroff, The obesity epidemic: the role of the National Institutes of Health, *Johns Hopkins Advanced Studies in Medicine,* 5(3), 122–123, March, 2005.

Part Five

Appendices

Appendix 1

The Heath-Carter Anthropometric Somatotype: Measurement and Assessment[1–4]

I. Equipment
   A. Weight scale
   B. Stadiometer
   C. Skinfold calipers
   D. Steel spreading or wooden sliding calipers
   E. Cloth or steel type
II. Body landmarks and measurement processes (Figure A1.1, Figure A1.2)
   A. Appropriate measurements are obtained from right side of body.
   B. Skinfold measures are replicated until within 5% limits, and skeletal measures are repeated until within 1% limits.
III. Skinfolds
   A. Taken between thumb and index finger and measurement is obtained approximately on centimeter below grasp with calipers.
   B. Triceps — midway between acromion and olecranon processes on the back of the upper arm with subject standing and arm extended downward (Figure A1.3).
   C. Subscapula — inferior angle of the scapula in parallel position to axilary border with the subject standing (Figure A1.3).
   D. Suprailiac — a few inches above and to the right of the anterior and superior spine of the iliac crest with subject standing (Figure A1.4).
   E. Calf — the medial side of the calf where maximal calf girth is located with subject sitting (Figure A1.4).

HEATH-CARTER SOMATOTYPE RATING FORM

NAME .... AGE .... SEX: M F NO: ....

OCCUPATION .... ETHNIC GROUP .... DATE ....

PROJECT: .... MEASURED BY: ....

Skinfolds mm

Triceps =

Subcapular =

Supraliac =

TOTAL SKINFOLDS = ☐

Calf =

TOTAL SKINFOLDS (mm)

Upper Limit	10.9	14.9	18.9	22.9	26.9	31.2	35.8	40.7	46.2	52.2	58.7	65.7	73.2	81.2	89.7	98.9	108.9	119.7	131.2	143.7	157.2	171.9	187.9	204.0
Mid-point	9.0	13.0	17.0	21.0	25.0	29.0	33.5	38.0	43.5	49.0	55.5	62.0	69.5	77.0	85.5	94.0	104.0	114.0	125.5	137.0	150.5	164.0	180.0	196.0
Lower Limit	7.0	11.0	15.0	19.0	23.0	27.0	31.3	35.9	40.8	46.3	52.3	58.8	65.8	73.3	81.3	89.8	99.0	109.0	119.8	131.3	143.8	157.3	172.0	188.0
FIRST COMPONENT	½	1	1½	2	2½	3	3½	4	4½	5	5½	6	6½	7	7½	8	8½	9	9½	10	10½	11	11½	12

Height cm ☐	139.7	143.5	147.3	151.1	154.9	158.8	162.6	166.4	170.2	174.0	177.6	181.6	165.4	189.2	193.0	196.9	200.7	204.5	208.3	212.1	215.9	219.7	223.5	227.3
Humeus width cm ☐	5.19	5.34	5.49	5.64	5.78	5.93	6.07	6.22	6.37	6.51	6.65	6.80	6.95	7.09	7.24	7.38	7.53	7.67	7.82	7.97	8.11	8.25	8.40	8.55
Femur width cm ☐	7.41	7.62	7.83	8.04	8.24	8.45	8.66	8.87	9.08	9.28	9.49	9.70	9.91	10.12	10.33	10.53	10.74	10.95	11.16	11.36	11.57	11.78	11.99	12.21
Biceps girth ☐ -T[a] ☐	23.7	24.4	25.0	25.7	26.3	27.0	27.7	28.3	29.0	29.7	30.3	31.0	31.6	32.2	33.0	33.6	34.3	35.0	35.6	36.3	37.0	37.6	38.3	39.0
Calf girth ☐ -C[a] ☐	27.7	28.5	29.3	30.1	30.8	31.6	32.4	33.2	33.9	34.7	35.5	36.3	37.1	37.8	38.6	39.4	40.2	41.0	41.7	42.5	43.3	44.1	44.9	45.6

SECOND COMPONENT	½	1	1½	2	2½	3	3½	4	4½	5	5½	6	6½	7	7½	8	8½	9

Weight kg =

Ht. / $\sqrt[3]{Wt.}$ = ☐

Upper Limit	39.65	40.74	41.43	42.13	42.82	43.48	44.18	44.84	45.53	46.23	46.92	47.58	48.25	48.94	49.63	50.33	50.99	51.68
Mid-point	and	40.20	41.09	41.79	42.48	43.14	43.84	44.50	45.19	45.89	46.32	47.24	47.94	48.60	49.29	49.99	50.68	51.34
Lower Limit	below	39.66	40.75	41.44	42.14	42.83	43.49	44.19	44.85	45.54	46.24	46.93	47.59	48.26	48.95	49.64	50.34	51.00
THIRD COMPONENT	½	1	1½	2	2½	3	3½	4	4½	5	5½	6	6½	7	7½	8	8½	9

	FIRST COMPONENT	SECOND COMPONENT	THIRD COMPONENT	
Anthropometric Somatotype				BY: ....
Anthropometric plus Photoscopic Somatotype				RATER:....................................

[a] Biceps girth in cm corrected for fat by subtracting triceps skinfold value expressed in cm,

[a] Calf girth in cm corrected for fat by subtracting medial calf skin fold cm.

FIGURE A1.1 Heath-Carter somatotype rating form. (From Carter, J.E.L. and B.H. Heath, *Somatotyping: Development and Applications,* 1990, Cambridge University Press, New York. Reprinted with the permission of Cambridge University Press.)

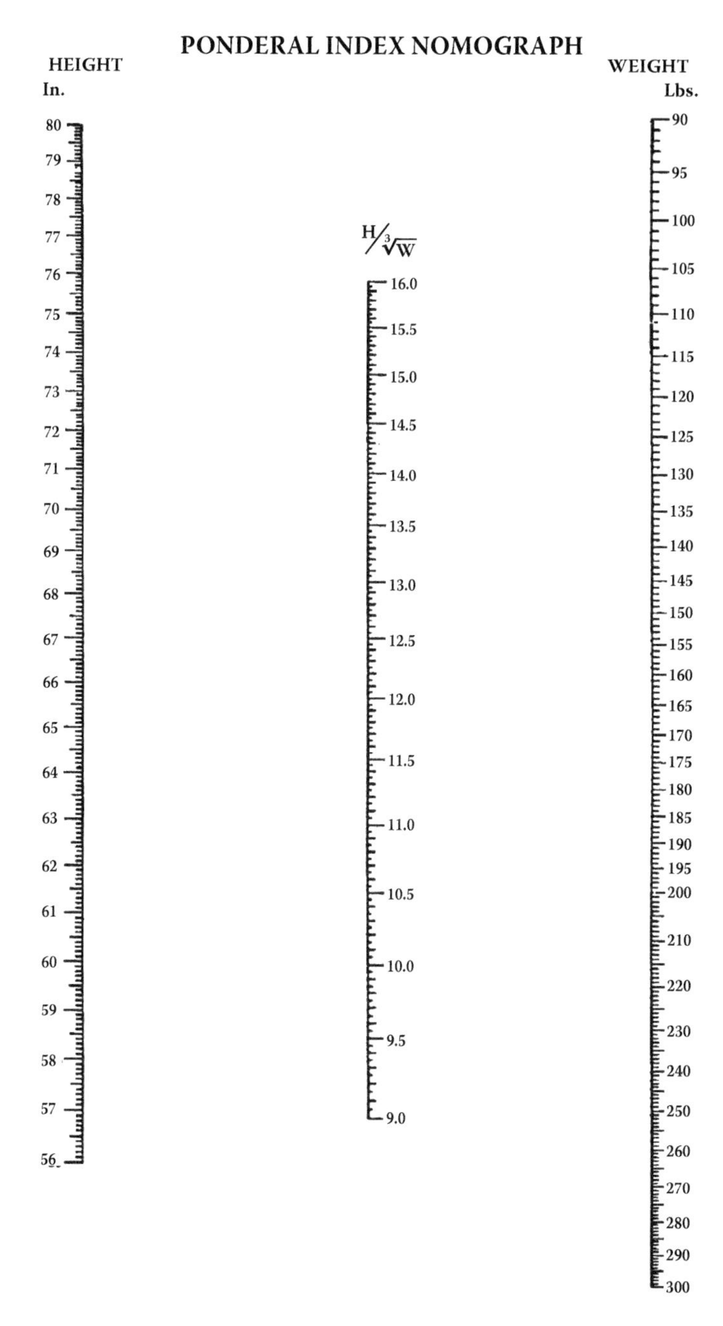

FIGURE A1.2 Ponderal index nonogram. (From Carter, J.E.L. and B.H. Heath, *Somatotyping: Development and Applications*, Cambridge University Press, New York. 1990. Reprinted with the permission of Cambridge University Press.)

Anthropometric Measurements

Triceps Skinfold

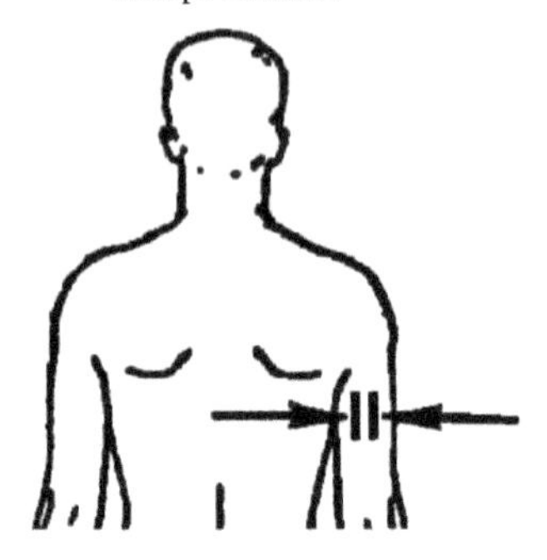

Subscapular Skinfold

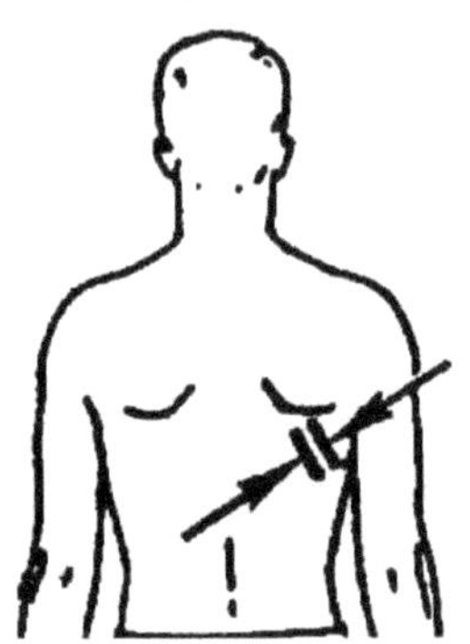

FIGURE A1.3 Anthropometric measurements. (From Churchill, E., J. McConville, L. Laubach, and R.R White, *Anthropometry of U. S. Army Aviators — 1970,* United States Soldier and Biological Chemical Command–Soldier Systems Center, Natick, MA, 1971. With permission.)

Anthropometric Measurements

Suprailiac Skinfold

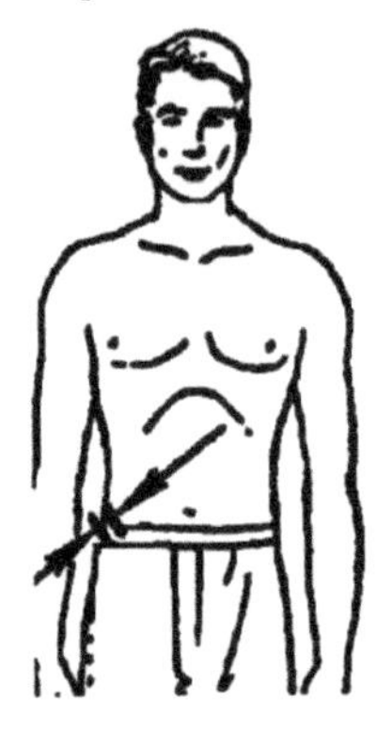

Medial Calf Skinfold

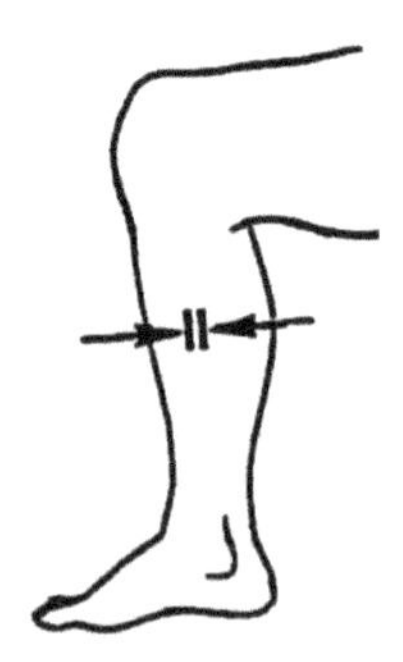

FIGURE A1.4 Anthropometric measurements. (From Churchill, E., J. McConville, L. Laubach, and R.R White, *Anthropometry of U. S. Army Aviators — 1970,* United States Soldier and Biological Chemical Command–Soldier Systems Center, Natick, MA, 1971. With permission.)

IV. Skeletal diameters
   A. Taken with enough pressure to compress tissue.
   B. Humerus — the medical and lateral condyles of the elbow with subject standing and right arm flexed upward to 90 degree angle (Figure A1.5).
   C. Femur — the medial and lateral processes of the right femur with subject sitting and leg bent at right angle (Figure A1.5).

Anthropometric Measurements

Elbow Breadth

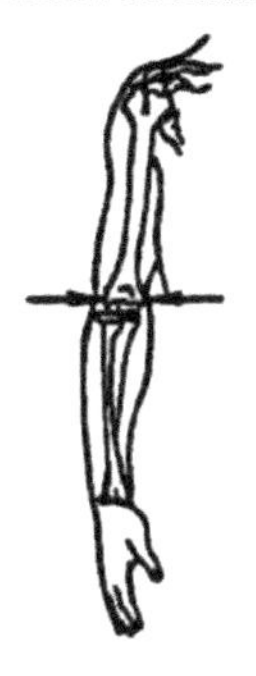

Knee Breadth

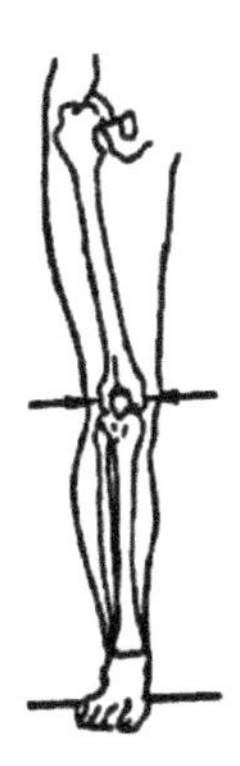

FIGURE A1.5 Anthropometric measurements. (From Churchill, E., J. McConville, L. Laubach, and R.R White, *Anthropometry of U. S. Army Aviators — 1970,* United States Soldier and Biological Chemical Command–Soldier Systems Center, Natick, MA, 1971. With permission.)

V. Body circumferences (Figure A1.6)
   A. Taken around landmark sites at right angles to the long axis of the body or body part.
   B. Biceps — midway between the shoulders and elbow with subject standing and arm flexed upward (Figure A1.6).
   C. Calf — at point of maximal circumferences of the calf muscle with subject standing (Figure A1.6).

Anthropometric Measurements

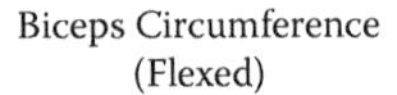

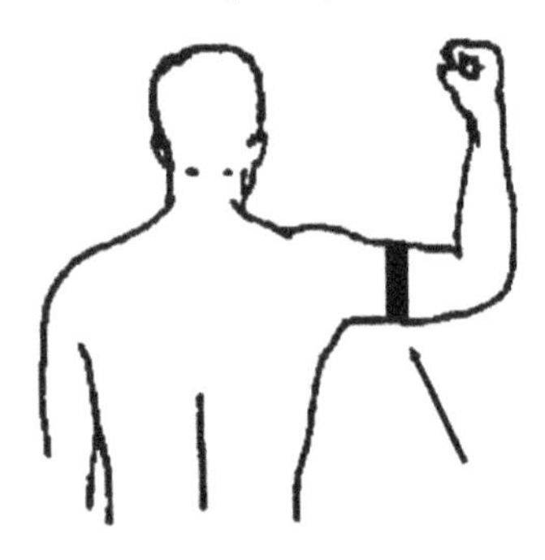

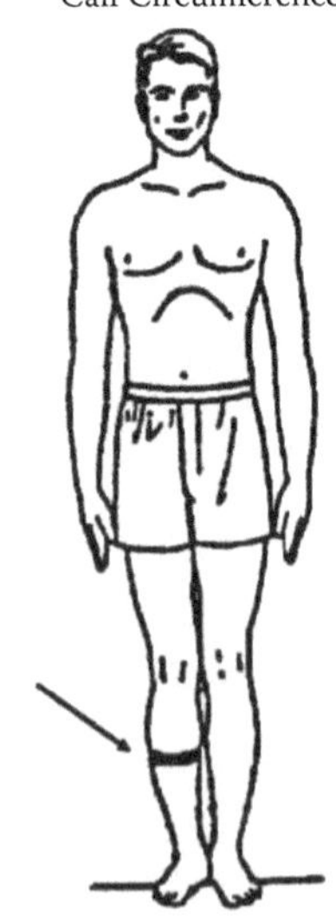

FIGURE A1.6 Anthropometric measurements. (From Churchill, E., J. McConville, L. Laubach, and R.R White, *Anthropometry of U. S. Army Aviators — 1970,* United States Soldier and Biological Chemical Command–Soldier Systems Center, Natick, MA, 1971. With permission.)

VI. Height and weight
  A. Height — measurement of body stature with subject standing.
  B. Weight — subject weighed on scale with minimal clothing.

VII. Endomorphy
  A. Record each of the skinfold measurements.
  B. Record sum of triceps, subscapular, and suprailiac skinfolds.
  C. Circle closest representative skinfold value in the lower to upper limit rating scale denoted by rows and columns on right.

VIII. Mesomorphy
  A. Record the height and each of the skeletal measurements.
  B. Correct biceps and calf circumference measurements by subtracting the respective skinfolds that have been converted from millimeters to centimeters (divide by 10).
  C. Record corrected bicep and calf measurements.
  D. Circle nearest height rating on scale.
  E. Circle nearest skeletal and circumference ratings for each of the measurements in the appropriate rows.
  F. Calculate average deviations of the measurements from the circled height designation. Column designations to the right of the height measure are termed to be positive, while designations to the left are termed to be negative.
  G. Utilize formula to find mesomorphic rating: 4.0 ($1/8 \times D$).
  H. Equals sum of column number deviations from height now.
  I. Circle mesomorphic rating (second component) based on obtained formula designation.

IX. Ectomorphy
  A. Record weight.
  B. Utilize Ponderal index nomograph to obtain height divided by the cube root of weight ratio.
  C. Circle closest representative ratio value in the lower to upper limit rating scale denoted by rows and columns on right.
  D. Circle ectomorphic rating (third component) directly under circled ratio value.

X. Decimalized anthropometric somatotype equations[3]
  A. Endomorphy:

  $\text{Endomorphy} = 0.7182 + 0.1451(x) - 0.00068(x^2) + 0.0000014(x^3)$.
  x = Sum of triceps, subscapular and supraspinale skinfolds. for height corrected endomorphy, multiply x by 170.18/height in cm.

  B. Mesomorphy:

  $\text{Mesomorphy} = [(0.858 \times \text{humerus breadth}) + (0.601 \times \text{femur breadth}) + (0.188 \times \text{corrected arm girth}) + (0.161 \times \text{corrected calf girth})] - (\text{height} \times 0.131) + 4.50$.

  C. Ectomorphy:

  $\text{Ectomorphy} = \text{HWR} \times 0.732 - 28.58$.

If HWR is less than 40.75 but more than 38.25:
Ectomorphy = HWR × 0.436 – 17.36.
If HWR is equal to or less than 38.25, give a rating of 0.1.
HWR = Height/cube root of weight.

REFERENCES

1. Carter, J.E.L., The Heath-Carter, *Somatotype Method,* 3rd ed., San Diego State University, San Diego, CA, 1980.
2. Hebbelinck, M. and W.D. Ross. Body type and performance, in *Fitness, Health, and Work Capacity: International Standards for Assessment,* Larson, L.A., Ed., Macmillan Publishing Co., New York, 1977.
3. Carter, J.E.L. and B.H. Heath, *Somatotyping: Development and Applications,* Cambridge University Press, New York, 1990.
4. Duquet, W. and J. E. L. Carter, Somatotyping. in *Kinantropometry and Exercise Physiology Laboratory Manual: Tests, Procedures, and Data,* 2nd ed. Vol. 1, Anthropometry, Eston, R.G. and T. Reilly, Eds., Routledge, London, June, 2001.

Appendix 2

Dysplasia Types and Subtypes: Measurement and Assessment[1,2]

I. Equipment
   A. Stadiometer
   B. Steel spreading or wooden sliding calipers
II. Body landmarks and measurement processes
   A. Upper trunk and upper limbs
      1. Biacromial breadth — the lateral projections of the acromial processes with subject standing.
      2. Chest breadth — at the level of the fifth to sixth ribs along the chest line with the subject standing.
      3. Elbow breadth — the medial and lateral condyles of both elbows with subject standing and arm flexed upward to 90 degree angle.
      4. Wrist breadth — the radial and ulna styloid processes of both wrists with subject standing and arms extended.
   B. Lower trunk and lower limbs
      1. Bi-iliac breadth — the iliac crests with subject standing.
      2. Bi-trochanteric breadth — the lateral projections of the trochanters with subject standing.
      3. Knee breadth — the heads of the tibia and fibula below knee level with subject sitting and legs bent at right angles.
      4. Ankle breadth — the malleoli of both ankles with subject standing
III. Dysplasia assessment
   A. All of the measurements are taken in centimeters and recorded on the data form (Figure A2.1). Height is obtained in inches and then converted to centimeters. The skeletal breadth is replicated until within 1% limits.

DYSPLASIA ANTHROPOMETRIC DATA

UPPER TRUNK AND ARMS		LOWER TRUNK AND LEGS	
Bi-acromial	______	Bi-iliac	______
Chest	______	Bi-trochanteric	______
Elbow (R)	______	Knee (R)	______
Elbow (L)	______	Knee (L)	______
Wrist (R)	______	Ankle (R)	______
Wrist (L)	______	Ankle (L)	______

Dysplasia Formulas

Upper Body

$$\text{Upper Trunk} + \text{Arms} = \frac{\text{Height}}{\text{Bi-acromial} + \text{Chest} + \text{Both Elbows} + \text{Both Wrists}}$$

Lower Body

$$\text{Lower Trunk} + \text{Legs} = \frac{\text{Height}}{\text{Bi-iliac} + \text{Bi-trochanteric} + \text{Both Knees} + \text{Both Ankles}}$$

Dysplasia Type

Upper Body	Lower Body
______	______

FIGURE A2.1 Dysplasia anthropometric data. (From Battinelli, T.A., *British Journal of Sports Medicine,* 18, 22–25, 1984. With permission from the BMJ Publishing Group.)

B. Calculate height/breadth ratios through the utilization of designated formulas on data form.
C. Type and subtype dysplasia classifications are determined by individual index deviation from group mean and standard deviation index scores (Figure A2.2 and Figure A2.3).

Classification of Dysplasia into Types (Letters and Subtypes (Symbols) on the Basis of Direction and Extent of Upper Trunk and Arms and Lower Trunk and Legs Relative to Mean and Standard Deviation Units.

Upper Truck and Arms				
	B--/B--	B--/B-	B--/L+	B--/L++
- 2 S.D. Units				
	B-/B--	B-/B-	B-/L+	B-/L++
Mean				
	L+/B--	L+/B-	L+/L+	L+/L++
+ 2 S.D. Units				
	L++/B--	L++/B-	L++/L+	L++/L++
	- 2 S.D. Units		Mean	+ 2 S.D. Units

Lower Truck and Legs

Key

Upper Trunk and Arms/Lower Trunk and Legs
B = Breadth predominance relative to length (direction)
L = Length predominance relative to breadth (direction)
+ or - = Slight predominance (extent)
S.D. = Standard Deviation

FIGURE A2.2 Classification of dysplasia into types (letters) and subtypes (symbols) on the basis of direction and extent of upper trunk and lower trunk and legs relative to mean and standard deviation units. From Battinelli, T.A., *British Journal of Sports Medicine,* 18, 22–25, 1984. With permission from the BMJ Publishing Group.)

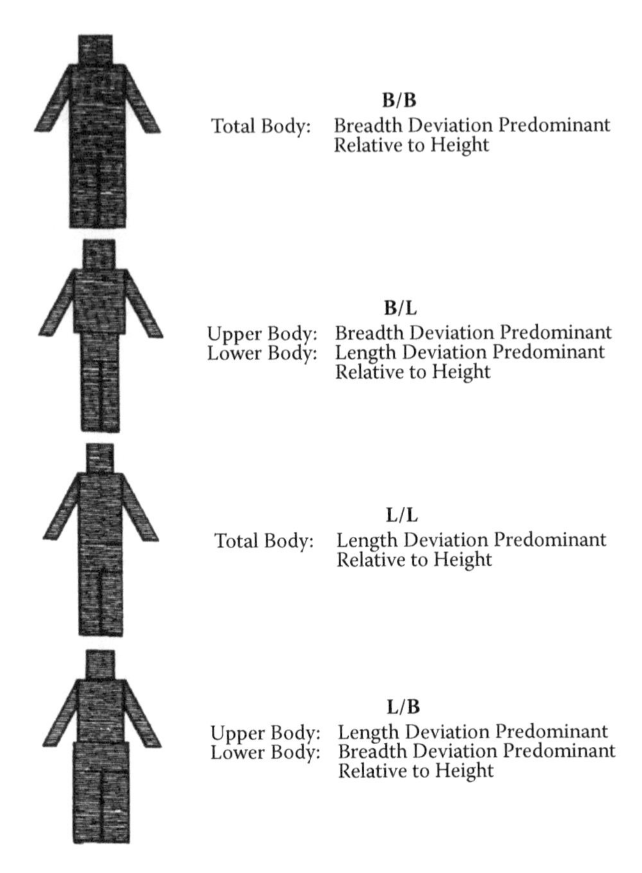

FIGURE A2.3 Dysplasia type representations. (From Battinelli, T.A., *British Journal of Sports Medicine,* 18, 22–25, 1984. With permission from the BMJ Publishing Group.)

REFERENCES

1. Battinelli, T.A., Simplistic approach to structural dysplasia assessment: description and validation, British Journal of Sports Medicine, 18, 22–25, 1984.
2. Behnke, A.R. and J.N. Wilmore, Evaluation and Regulation of Body Build and Composition, Prentice-Hall Inc., Englewood Cliff, NJ, 1974.

Appendix 3

Body Composition: Measurement and Assessment[1–4]

I. Equipment — skinfold calipers

II. Body landmarks and measurements processes (Figure A3.1)
   - A. Selective measurements are taken from right side of body and are replicated until within 5%.
   - B. Appropriate skinfold is taken between thumb and index finger, and measurement is obtained approximately one centimeter below grasp with calipers.

III. Male (Figure A3.2)
   - A. Chest — at the midway point between the anterior fold and the axilla and the chest line.
   - B. Abdomen — horizontally to the right of the umbilicus.
   - C. Thigh — the vertical fold on the front of the thigh midway between hip and knee.

IV. Female (Figure A3.3)
   - A. Triceps — midway between acromion and olecranon processes on the back of the upper arm.
   - B. Thigh — the vertical fold on the front of the thigh midway between hip and knee.
   - C. Supralium — at the midaxillary line of the iliac crest.

V. Nomogram use (Figure A3.1)
   - A. Record measurements.
   - B. Insert age in years and the sum of the three measurements on the nomogram.
   - C. Read appropriate percent body fat figure from chart.

VI. Fat and fat free body weight (Figure A3.4)
   - A. Total weight × present fat = fat body weight
   - B. Total weight – fat body weight = fat free body weight (Figure A3.5).

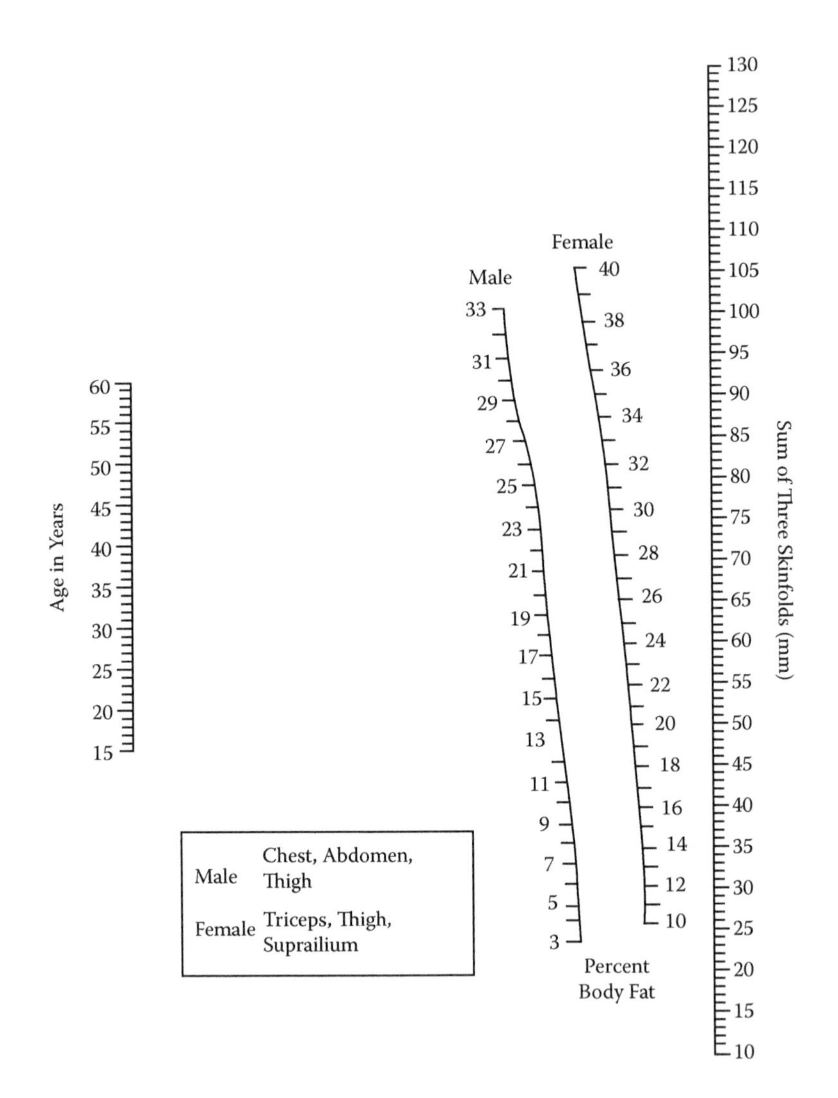

FIGURE A3.1 Nomogram for the estimation of body fat. (From Baun, W. B., M. R. Baun, and P. B. Raven, *Research Quarterly for Exercise and Sport,* 52, 380–384, 1981. With the permission of the American Alliance for Health, Physical Education, Recreation, and Dance.)

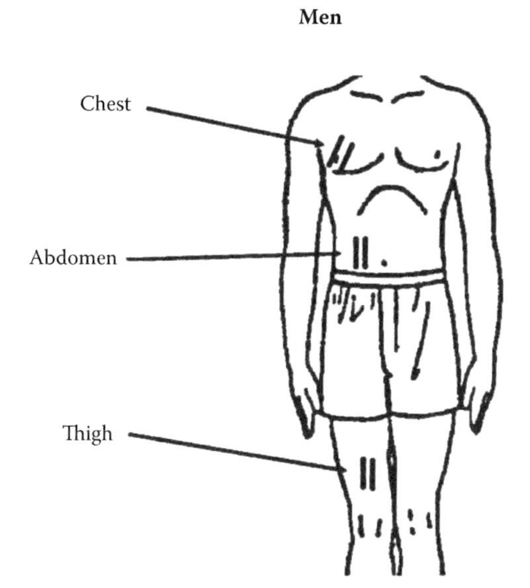

FIGURE A3.2 Body composition measurements, men. (Adapted from Churchill, E., J. McConville, L. Laubach, and R.R White, *Anthropometry of U. S. Army Aviators — 1970,* United States Soldier and Biological Chemical Command–Soldier Systems Center, Natick, MA, 1971. With permission.)

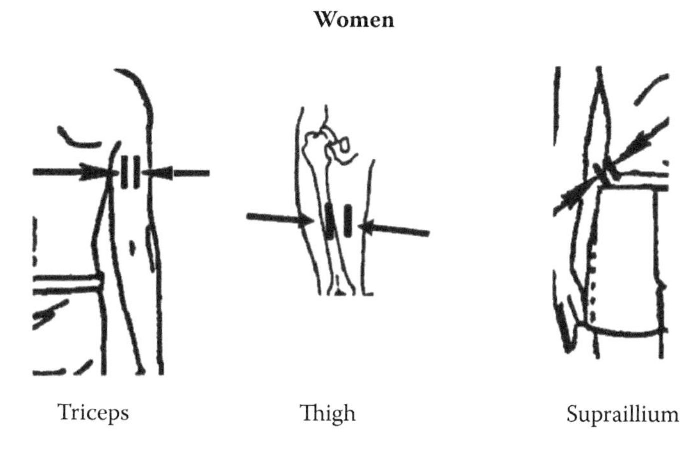

FIGURE A3.3 Body composition measurements, women. (Adapted from Churchill, E., J. McConville, L. Laubach, and R.R White, *Anthropometry of U. S. Army Aviators — 1970,* United States Soldier and Biological Chemical Command–Soldier Systems Center, Natick, MA, 1971. With permission.)

Body Composition: Percent Fat Classifications

	PERCENT BODY FAT	
CLASSIFICATION	MEN	WOMEN
Very lean	<=10	<=12
Lean	11-14	15-19
Average	15-18	20-24
Fat	19-23	25-31
Overfat (obese)	>=24	>=32

FIGURE A3.4 Body composition: percent fat classifications. (From Brown, H. L., *Lifetime Fitness,* 4th ed., Allyn and Bacon, Boston, 1986. Reprinted with permission from Pearson Education.)

Body Composition

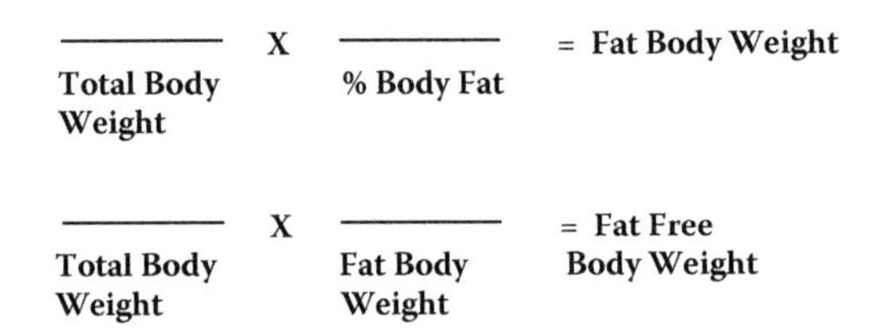

FIGURE A3.5 Body composition.

REFERENCES

1. Brown, H.L., *Lifetime Fitness,* 4th ed., Allyn and Bacon, Boston, 1986.
2. Churchill, E., J. McConville, L. Laubach, and R.R White, *Anthropometry of U. S. Army Aviators — 1970,* United States Soldier and Biological Chemical Command–Soldier Systems Center, Natick, MA, 1971.
3. Jackson, A.A. and M.L. Pollock, Generalized equations for predicting body density of men, *British Journal of Nutrition,* 40, 497–504, 1978.
4. Jackson, A.A., M.L. Pollock, and A. Ward, Generalized equation for predicting body density of women, *Medicine and Science in Sports and Exercise,* 12, 175–182, 1980.

Appendix 4

Resistance Exercises: Free Weights

I. Front curls (Figure A4.1, Figure A4.2, Figure A4.3, Figure A4.4)
   A. Standing position
   B. Bar resting in front of thighs
   C. Underhand grip (shoulder width)
   D. Pull weight upward by flexing arms at elbows to chest and return to starting position.

Muscle Strength and Muscle Endurance Tests

Ratings	Grip Strength		Sit-Ups		Push-Ups	Modified Push-Ups
	Men	Women	Men	Women		
Good	136>	81>	41>	36>	36>	31>
Fair	100-135	55-80	30-40	25-35	25-35	20-30
Low	<99	<54	<29	<24	<24	<19

FIGURE A4.1 Muscle strength and muscle endurance tests. (From Seiger, L., K. Vanderpool, and D. Barnes, *Fitness and Wellness Strategies,* 1995. With permission from the McGraw-Hill Companies.)

Modified Sit and Reach Test

Ratings	Men	Women
	Sit & Reach	
Good	10+	10+>
Fair	6-9	6-9
Low	<6	<6

FIGURE A4.2 Modified sit and reach test. From Seiger, L., K. Vanderpool, and D. Barnes, *Fitness and Wellness Strategies,* 1995. With permission from the McGraw-Hill Companies.)

Muscle Strength, Muscle Endurance, and Flexibility Tests

Name ____

	Score	**Percentile Level**
Grip Strength	_____	_____
Sit-ups	_____	_____
Push-ups	_____	_____
Modified Push-ups	_____	_____
Sit and Reach	_____	_____

FIGURE A4.3 Muscle strength, muscle endurance, and flexibility tests.

II. Reverse curls
   A. Standing position
   B. Bar resting in front of thighs.
   C. Overhand grip (shoulder width)
   D. Pull weight upward flexing arms at elbows to chest and return to starting position.
III. Upright rowing motions
   A. Standing position
   B. Bar resting in front of thighs
   C. Overhand grip (shoulder width)
   D. Pull weight upward with elbows in an outward position, close to front of body, to neck.
IV. Shoulder Press
   A. Standing position.
   B. Bar resting on upper chest at shoulder level
   C. Overhand grip (shoulder width)
   D. Push weight upward by straightening arms over head and return to starting position.
V. Half squats
   A. Standing position
   B. Bar resting on back of shoulders
   C. Wide overhand grip
   D. Feet flat on floor, with back in vertical position, bend knees to 90° angle and return to starting position

Weight Training Record

Name ________________________________

Exercise	Sets/Weights/Repetitions				

FIGURE A4.3 Weight training record.

VI. Pullovers
- A. Lying position on back and on bench
- B. Feet flat on floor
- C. Arms extended overhead grasping bar with overhand grip (shoulder width)
- D. Pull weight upward and overhead to chest and return to starting position.

VII. Prone press
- A. Lying on back on bench
- B. Feet flat on floor or on bench
- C. Bar resting on chest
- D. Overhand grip (shoulder width)
- E. Push weight upward by straightening arms and return to starting position.

VIII. Dips
- A. Body in cross rest position (vertical) with hands gripping pommels or bars and arms straight.

  B. Dip downward bending arms at elbows to 90° angle, keeping body straight, and return to starting position.

IX. Sit-ups
  A. Lying on back on abdominal board with feet placed in stirrups, knees bent, and arms crossed in front of chest.
  B. Curl head, neck, and back upward toward knees and return to starting position.

X. Pushups
  A. Lying on stomach on mat
  B. Hands placed on mat just outside shoulders and chest with body in straight alignment and knees on floor, straighten arms and return to starting position.

XI. Modified pushups
  A. Lying on stomach on mat
  B. Hands placed on mat just outside shoulders and chest with body in a straight alignment and knees on floor, straighten arms and return to starting position

XII. Safety precautions
  A. Do not lock joints under weight resistance.
  B. Do no compress spinal vertebrae of lower back in arched position under weight resistance.

Appendix 5

Aerobic and Anaerobic Conditioning: Assessment and Classification

- Sample walking program (Figure A5.1)

A Sample Walking Program

During each week of the program, try to walk briskly at least 5 days per week. Always start with a 5-minute, slower-paced walk to warm up, and end with a 5-minute, slower-paced walk to cool down. (Warm-up and cool-down sessions totaling 10 minutes are included in the "total time" column.) As you walk, check your pulse periodically to see whether you're moving within your target heart rate zone.

Week	Warm up	Target zone	Cool down	Total time
Week 1	Walk 5 min.	Walk briskly 5 min.	Walk 5 min.	15 min.
Week 2	Walk 5 min.	Walk briskly 7 min.	Walk 5 min.	17 min.
Week 3	Walk 5 min.	Walk briskly 9 min.	Walk 5 min.	19 min.
Week 4	Walk 5 min.	Walk briskly 11 min.	Walk 5 min.	21 min.
Week 5	Walk 5 min.	Walk briskly 13 min.	Walk 5 min.	23 min.
Week 6	Walk 5 min.	Walk briskly 15 min.	Walk 5 min.	25 min.
Week 7	Walk 5 min.	Walk briskly 18 min.	Walk 5 min.	28 min.
Week 8	Walk 5 min.	Walk briskly 20 min.	Walk 5 min.	30 min.
Week 9	Walk 5 min.	Walk briskly 23 min.	Walk 5 min.	33 min.
Week 10	Walk 5 min.	Walk briskly 26 min.	Walk 5 min.	36 min.
Week 11	Walk 5 min.	Walk briskly 28 min.	Walk 5 min.	38 min.
Week 12	Walk 5 min.	Walk briskly 30 min.	Walk 5 min.	40 min.
Week 13 on:	Walk 5 min.	Continue. (See below.)	Walk 5 min.	

As you become more fit, try to walk within the upper range of your target zone. Gradually increase your brisk walking time from 30 to 60 minutes, most days of the week. Enjoy the outdoors!

FIGURE A5.1 A sample walking program. (From Your Guide to Physical Activity and Your Heart, National Institutes of Health, National Heart, Lung, and Blood Institute, NIH Publication No. 06-5714, June, 2006.)

- Sample jogging program (Figure A5.2)

A Sample Jogging Program

During each week of the program, try to jog at least 5 days per week. For your warm up, walk for 5 minutes. For your cool down, walk for 3 minutes and then stretch for 2 minutes more. (Warm-up and cool-down sessions totaling 10 minutes are included in the "total time" column.) As you jog, check your pulse periodically to see whether you're moving within your target heart rate zone. If you're over 40 and haven't been active in a while, begin with the walking program. After you complete the walking program, start with Week 3 of the jogging program.

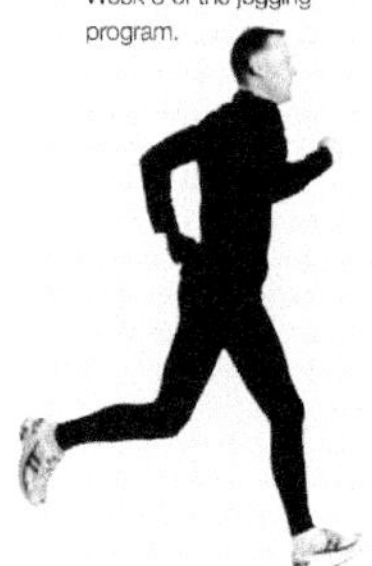

Week	Warm up	Jogging in your target zone	Cool down	Total time
Week 1	Walk 5 min., then stretch	Walk 10 min. Try to walk without stopping.	Walk 3 min., stretch 2 min.	20 min.
Week 2	Walk 5 min., then stretch	Walk 5 min., jog 1 min., walk 5 min., jog 1 min.	Walk 3 min., stretch 2 min.	22 min.
Week 3	Walk 5 min., then stretch	Walk 5 min., jog 3 min., walk 5 min., jog 3 min.	Walk 3 min., stretch 2 min.	26 min.
Week 4	Walk 5 min., then stretch	Walk 4 min., jog 5 min., walk 4 min., jog 5 min.	Walk 3 min., stretch 2 min.	28 min.
Week 5	Walk 5 min., then stretch	Walk 4 min., jog 5 min., walk 4 min., jog 5 min.	Walk 3 min., stretch 2 min.	28 min.
Week 6	Walk 5 min., then stretch	Walk 4 min., jog 6 min., walk 4 min., jog 6 min.	Walk 3 min., stretch 2 min.	30 min.
Week 7	Walk 5 min., then stretch	Walk 4 min., jog 7 min., walk 4 min., jog 7 min.	Walk 3 min., stretch 2 min.	32 min.
Week 8	Walk 5 min., then stretch	Walk 4 min., jog 8 min., walk 4 min., jog 8 min.	Walk 3 min., stretch 2 min.	34 min.
Week 9	Walk 5 min., then stretch	Walk 4 min., jog 9 min., walk 4 min., jog 9 min.	Walk 3 min., stretch 2 min.	36 min.
Week 10	Walk 5 min., then stretch	Walk 4 min., jog 13 min.	Walk 3 min., stretch 2 min.	27 min.
Week 11	Walk 5 min., then stretch	Walk 4 min., jog 15 min.	Walk 3 min., stretch 2 min.	29 min.
Week 12	Walk 5 min., then stretch	Walk 4 min., jog 17 min.	Walk 3 min., stretch 2 min.	31 min.
Week 13	Walk 5 min., then stretch	Walk 2 min., jog slowly 2 min., jog 17 min.	Walk 3 min., stretch 2 min.	31 min.
Week 14	Walk 5 min., then stretch	Walk 1 min., jog slowly 3 min., jog 17 min.	Walk 3 min., stretch 2 min.	31 min.
Week 15	Walk 5 min., then stretch	Jog slowly 3 min., jog 17 min.	Walk 3 min., stretch 2 min.	30 min.
Week 16 on:	Walk 5 min., then stretch	Continue. (See below.)	Walk 3 min., stretch 2 min.	

As you become more fit, try to jog within the upper range of your target zone. Gradually, increase your jogging time from 20 to 30 minutes (or up to 60 minutes, if you wish). Keep track of your goals—and keep on enjoying yourself.

FIGURE A5.2 A sample jogging program. (From Your Guide to Physical Activity and Your Heart, National Institutes of Health, National Heart, Lung, and Blood Institute, NIH Publication No. 06-5714, June, 2006.)

- 1 1/2-Mile run (Figure A5.3)

Time (min:sec)	Estimated VO_{2max}
7:30 and under	75
7:31–8:00	72
8:01–8:30	67
8:31–9:00	62
9:01–9:30	58
9:31–10:00	55
10:01–10:30	52
10:31–11:00	49
11:01–11:30	46
11:31–12:00	44
12:01–12:30	41
12:31–13:00	39
13:01–13:30	37
13:31–14:00	36
14:01–14:30	34
14:31–15:00	33
15:01–15:30	31
15:31–16:00	30
16:01–16:30	28
16:31–17:00	27
17:01–17:30	26
17:31–18:00	25

FIGURE A5.3 Estimated VO_{2max} from 1.5-mile run time. (From Wilmore, J.H. and J.A. Bergfeld, in *Sports Medicine and Physiology,* Strauss, R.H., Ed., W.B. Saunders Company, Philadelphia, 1979. With permission from Elsevier.)

- Exercise target zones (Figure A5.4)

Age	Target Heart Rate Zone 50/70 – 85%	Maximum Heart Rates
20	100/140 – 170	200
25	98/137 – 166	195
30	95/133 – 162	190
35	93/130 – 157	185
40	90/136 – 153	180
45	88/123 – 149	175
50	85/119 – 145	170
55	83/116 – 139	165
60	80/112 – 136	160
65	78/108 – 132	155
70	75/105 – 128	150

Formula Utilization - 220 – Age = Maximum Heart Rate

FIGURE A5.4 Maximal and submaximal heart rates and target zones for different age levels. (Adapted from Your Guide to Physical Activity and Your Heart, National Institutes of Health, National Heart, Lung, and Blood Institute, NIH Publication No. 06-5714, June, 2006.)

- Classification of physical activity intensity (Figure A5.5)

	Endurance-type activity								Strength-type exercise
	Relative intensity			Absolute intensity (METs) in healthy adults (age in years)					Relative intensity*
Intensity	**$\dot{V}O_2$ max (%) heart rate reserve (%)**	**Maximal heart rate (%)**	**RPE†**	**Young (20–39)**	**Middle-aged (40–64)**	**Old (65–79)**	**Very old (80+)**	**RPE**	**Maximal voluntary contraction (%)**
Very light	<25	<30	<9	<3.0	<2.5	<2.0	≤1.25	<10	<30
Light	25–44	30–49	9–10	3.0–4.7	2.5–4.4	2.0–3.5	1.26–2.2	10–11	30–49
Moderate	45–59	50–69	11–12	4.8–7.1	4.5–5.9	3.6–4.7	2.3–2.95	12–13	50–69
Hard	60–84	70–89	13–16	7.2–10.1	6.0–8.4	4.8–6.7	3.0–4.25	14–16	70–84
Very hard	≥85	≥90	>16	≥10.2	≥8.5	≥6.8	≥4.25	17–19	>85
Maximal‡	100	100	20	12.0	10.0	8.0	5.0	20	100

Table 2-4 provided courtesy of Haskell and Pollock.

*Based on 8–12 repetitions for persons under age 50 years and 10–15 repetitions for persons aged 50 years and older.

†Borg rating of Relative Perceived Exertion 6–20 scale (Borg 1982).

‡Maximal values are mean values achieved during maximal exercise by healthy adults. Absolute intensity (METs) values are approximate mean values for men. Mean values for women are approximately 1–2 METs lower than those for men.

FIGURE A5.5 Classification of physical activity intensity based on physical activity lasting up to sixty minutes. (From Physical Activity and Health: A Report of the Surgeon General, United States Department of Health and Human Services, 1996. With permission.)

- Cardiovascular endurance (Figure A5.6)

Cardiovascular Endurance

Name ____________________________________

	Relative Intensity (Percent of Maximum Heart Rate)	Rating of Perceived Exertion	Absolute Intensity
Walking/ Jogging	______________	__________	__________
Mile and a Half Run*	______________	__________	__________

***VO_{2max} can be divided by 3.5 to equal MET Absolute Intensity Rating**

FIGURE A5.6 Cardiovascular endurance.

- Walking/jogging record (Figure A5.7)

Jogging Record

Name ______________________________

Date	Heart Rate (Resting)	Distance Run/ Walk	Heart Rate (Exercise)	Time	RPE	Heart Rate Recovery

Heart Rates
Resting: Prior to Activity
Exercise: Immediate End of Exercise
Recovery: Two Minutes after Cessation of Exercise
RPE – Rate of Perceived Exertion

FIGURE A5.7 Jogging record.

Appendix 6

Nutrition Guidelines

- Estimated daily calorie needs (Figure A6.1)

Estimated Daily Calorie Needs

To determine which food intake pattern to use for an individual, the following chart gives an estimate of individual calorie needs. The calorie range for each age/sex group is based on physical activity level, from sedentary to active.

	Calorie Range		
Children	Sedentary	→	Active
2–3 years	1,000	→	1,400
Females			
4–8 years	1,200	→	1,800
9–13	1,600	→	2,200
14–18	1,800	→	2,400
19–30	2,000	→	2,400
31–50	1,800	→	2,200
51+	1,600	→	2,200
Males			
4–8 years	1,400	→	2,000
9–13	1,800	→	2,600
14–18	2,200	→	3,200
19–30	2,400	→	3,000
31–50	2,200	→	3,000
51+	2,000	→	2,800

Sedentary means a lifestyle that includes only the light physical activity associated with typical day-to-day life.

Active means a lifestyle that includes physical activity equivalent to walking more than 3 miles per day at 3 to 4 miles per hour, in addition to the light physical activity associated with typical day-to-day life.

FIGURE A6.1 Estimated daily calorie needs. (From *Dietary Guidelines for Americans, 2005*, 6th ed., United States Department of Agriculture, Center for Nutrition Policy and Promotion, April, 2005.)

- Dietary goals (Figure A6.2)

Macronutrient	Range (percent of energy)		
	Children, 1–3 y	Children, 4–18 y	Adults
Fat	30–40	25–35	20–35
n-6 polyunsaturated fatty acids[a] (linoleic acid)	5–10	5–10	5–10
n-3 polyunsaturated fatty acids[a] (α-linolenic acid)	0.6–1.2	0.6–1.2	0.6–1.2
Carbohydrate	45–65	45–65	45–65
Protein	5–20	10–30	10–35

[a] Approximately 10% of the total can come from longer-chain *n*-3 or *n*-6 fatty acids.

FIGURE A6.2 Dietary reference intakes: acceptable macronutrient distribution ranges. (From *Dietary Reference Intakes for Energy, Carbohydrates, Fiber, Fat, Fatty Acids, Cholesterol, Protein, and Amino Acids,* Food and Nutrition Board, Institute of Medicine, The National Academies, Washington, DC, 2002. With permission.)

- Dietary guidelines (Figure A6.3 and Figure A6.4)

Macronutrient	Recommendation
Dietary cholesterol	As low as possible while consuming a nutritionally adequate diet
Trans fatty acids	As low as possible while consuming a nutritionally adequate diet
Saturated fatty acids	As low as possible while consuming a nutritionally adequate diet
Added sugars	Limit to no more than 25% of total energy

FIGURE A6.3 Dietary reference intakes. Additional macronutrient recommendations. (From *Dietary Reference Intakes for Energy, Carbohydrates, Fiber, Fat, Fatty Acids, Cholesterol, Protein, and Amino Acids,* Food and Nutrition Board, Institute of Medicine, The National Academies, Washington, DC, 2002. With permission.)

Dietary Guidelines for Americans 2005

Key Recommendations for the General Population

Adequate Nutrient within Calorie Needs

- Consume a variety of nutrient-dense foods and beverages within and among the basic food groups while choosing foods that limit the intake of saturated and *trans* fats, cholesterol, added sugars, salt, and alcohol.
- Meet recommended intakes within energy needs by adopting a balanced eating pattern, such as the U.S. Department of Agriculture (USDA) Food Guide or the Dietary Approaches to Stop Hypertension (DASH) Eating Plan.

Weight Management

- To maintain body weight in a healthy range, balance calories from foods and beverages with calories expended.
- To prevent gradual weight gain over time, make small decreases in food and beverage calories and increase physical activity.

Physical Activity

- Engage in regular physical activity and reduce sedentary activities to promote health, psychological well-being, and a healthy body weight.
  - To reduce the risk of chronic disease in adulthood: Engage in at least 30 minutes of moderate-intensity physical activity, abov e usual activity, at work or home on most days of the week.
  - For most people, greater health benefits can be obtained by engaging in physical acitivity of more vigorous intensity or longer duration.
  - To hel manage body weight and prevent gradual, unhealthy body weight gain in adulthood: Engage in approximately 60 minutes of moderate- to vigorous-intensity activity on most days of the week while not exceeding caloric intake requirements.
  - To sustain weight loss in adulthood: Participate in at least 60 to 90 minutes of daily moderate-intensity physical activity while not exceeding caloric intake requirements. Some people may need to consult with a healthcare provider before participating in this level of activity.
- Achieve physical fitness by including cardiovascular conditioning, stretching exercises for flexibility, and resistance exercises or calisthenics for muscle strength and endurance.

Food Groups to Encourage

- Consume a sufficient amount of fruits and vegetables while staying within energy needs. Two cups of fruit and 2 1/2 cups of vegetables per day are recommeded for a reference 2,000-calorie intake, with higher or lower amounts depending on the calorie level.
- Choose a variety of fruits and vegetables each day. In particular, select from all five vegetable subgroups (dark green, orange, legumes, starchy vegetables, and other vegetables) several times a week.
- Consume 3 or more ounce-equivalents of whole-grain products per day, with the rest of the recommended grains coming from enriched or whole-grain products. In general, at least half the grains should come from whole grains.
- Consume 3 cups per day of fat-free or low-fat milk or equivalent milk products.

Fats

- Consume less than 10 percent of calories from saturated fatty acids and less than 300 mg/day of cholesterol, and keep *trans* fatty acid consumption as low as possible.
- Keep total fat intake between 20 to 35 percent of calories, with most fats coming from sources of polyunsaturated and monounsaturated fatty acids, such as fish, nuts, and vegetable oils.

FIGURE A6.4 Dietary guidelines for Americans 2005. (From *Dietary Guidelines for Americans, 2005*, 6th ed., United States Department of Agriculture, Center for Nutrition Policy and Promotion, April, 2005.)

Continued.

- When selecting and preparing meat, poultry, dry beans, and milk or milk products, make choices that are lean, low-fat, or fat-free.
- Limit intake of fats and oils high in saturated and/or *trans* fatty acids, and choose products low in such fats and oils.

Carbohydrates
- Choose fiber-rich fruits, vegetables, and whole grains often.
- Choose and prepare foods and beverages with little added sugars or caloric sweeteners, such as amounts suggested by the USDA Food Guide and the DASH Eating Plan.
- Reduce the incidence of dental caries by practicing good oral hygiene and consuming sugar- and starch-containing foods and beverages less frequently.

Sodium and Potassium
- Consume less than 2,300 mg (approximately 1 teaspoon of salt) of sodium per day.
- Choose and prepare foods with little salt. At the same time, consume potassium-rich foods, such as fruits and vegetables.

Alcoholic Beverages
- Those who choose to drink alcoholic beverages should do so sensibly and in moderation — defined as the consumption of up to one drink per day for women and up to two drinks per day for men.
- Alcoholic beverages should not be consumed by some individuals, including those who cannot restrict their alcohol intake, women of childbearing age who may become pregnant, pregnant and lactating women, children and adolescents, individuals taking medications that can interact with alcohol, and those with specific medical conditions.
- Alcoholic beverages should be avoided by individuals engaging in activities that require attention, skill, or coordination, such as driving or operating machinery.

Food Safety
- To avoid microbial foodborne illness:
  - Clean hands, food contact surfaces, and fruits and vegetables. Meat and pountry should not be washed or rinsed.
  - Separate raw, cooked, and ready-to-eat foods while shopping, preparing, or storing foods.
  - Cook foods to a safe temperature to kill microorganisms.
  - Chill (refrigerate) perishable food promptly and defrost foods properly.
  - Avoid raw (unpasteurized) milk or any products made from unpasteurized milk, raw or partially cooked eggs or foods containing raw eggs, raw or undercooked meat and poultry, unpasteurized juices, and raw sprouts.

FIGURE A6.4 *Continued.*

- Food guide list (Figure A6.5)

Saturated Fat, Total Fat, Cholesterol, and Omega-3 Content of Meat, Fish, and Poultry in 3-Ounce Portions Cooked Without Added Fat

Source	Saturated Fat g/3 oz	Total Fat g/3 oz	Cholesterol mg/3 oz	Omega-3 g/3 oz
Lean Red Meats				
Beef (rump roast, shank, bottom round, sirloin)	1.4	4.2	71	—
Lamb (shank roast, sirloin roast, shoulder roast, loin chops, sirloin chops, center leg chop)	2.8	7.8	78	—
Pork (sirloin cutlet, loin roast, sirloin roast, center roast, butterfly chops, loin chops)	3.0	8.6	71	—
Veal (blade roast, sirloin chops, shoulder roast, loin chops, rump roast, shank)	2.0	4.9	93	—
Organ Meats				
Liver				
Beef	1.6	4.2	331	—
Calf	2.2	5.9	477	—
Chicken	1.6	4.6	537	—
Sweetbread	7.3	21.3	250	—
Kidney	0.9	2.9	329	—
Brains	2.5	10.7	1,747	—
Heart	1.4	4.8	164	—
Poultry				
Chicken (without skin)				
Light (roasted)	1.1	3.8	72	—
Dark (roasted)	2.3	8.3	71	—
Turkey (without skin)				
Light (roasted)	0.9	2.7	59	—
Dark (roasted)	2.0	6.1	72	—
Fish				
Haddock	0.1	0.8	63	0.22
Flounder	0.3	1.3	58	0.47
Salmon	1.7	7.0	54	1.88
Tuna, light, canned in water	0.2	0.7	25	0.24
Shellfish				
Crustaceans				
Lobster	0.1	0.5	61	0.07
Crab meat				
Alaskan King Crab	0.1	1.3	45	0.38
Blue Crab	0.2	1.5	85	0.45
Shrimp	0.2	0.9	166	0.28
Mollusks				
Abalone	0.3	1.3	144	0.15
Clams	0.2	1.7	57	0.33
Mussels	0.7	3.8	48	0.70
Oysters	1.3	4.2	93	1.06
Scallops	0.1	1.2	56	0.36
Squid	0.6	2.4	400	0.84

FIGURE A6.5 Saturated fat, cholesterol, and omega-3 content of meat, fish, and poultry in 3-ounce portions cooked without added fat food guide list. (From National Heart, Lung, and Blood Institute, *Third Report of the National Cholesterol Education Program (NCEP) Expert Panel on Detection, Evaluation, and Treatment of High Blood Cholesterol in Adults (Adult Treatment Panel III) Final Report,* National Institutes of Health, National Heart, Lung, and Blood Institute, NIH Publication No. 02-5215, September, 2002.)

- Vitamin and mineral guide lists (Figure A6.6 and Figure A6.7)

Vitamin	Functions	Food Sources
Fat-Soluble Vitamins		
Vitamin A	Maintains normal vision and healthy skin and mucous membranes; necessary for normal growth and for reproduction	Liver, butter, whole milk, egg yolks; margarine, skim milk, and certain breakfast cereals are fortified with vitamin A; the body also makes vitamin A from carotenoids, compounds present in dark-green leafy vegetables, yellow and orange vegetables, and fruit
Vitamin D	Promotes calcium and phosphorus absorption from the intestines; influences bone growth	Liver, butter, fatty fish, egg yolks; milk is fortified with vitamin D
Vitamin E	Antioxidant that prevents cells from being damaged by various biochemical reactions that occur naturally	Best sources are vegetable oils; also found in nuts, seeds, whole grains, and wheat germ
Vitamin K	Aids in blood clotting	Best source is dark-green leafy vegetables; also found in cereals, dairy products, meat, and fruits
Water-Soluble Vitamins		
Vitamin C	Promotes growth of connective tissues; antioxidant	Citrus fruits, tomatoes, broccoli, green peppers, strawberries, melons, cabbage, and leafy green vegetables; vitamin C is destroyed when foods are overcooked or cooked in large amounts of water
Thiamin (Vitamin B_1)	Aids in obtaining energy from carbohydrates	Meat, eggs, beans, and whole grains; enriched breads and cereals
Riboflavin (Vitamin B_2)	Aids in energy production and in many other biochemical processes	Liver, milk, and dark-green leafy vegetables; whole grains and enriched breads an cereals
Niacin	Aids in energy production from fats, proteins, and carbohydrates; aids in manufacture of fatty acids	Grain products, meat, poultry, fish, nuts, and beans
Pyridoxine (Vitamin B_6)	Aids in manufacture of amino acids; aids in energy production from protein	Meat, poultry, fish, grain products, and fruits and vegetables
Cobalamin (Vitamin B_{12})	Aids in DNA synthesis, and in energy production from fatty acids and carbohydrates; aids in production of amino acids	Meat, milk and milk products, and eggs
Folacin	Aids in manufacture of genetic material in cells; aids in production of amino acids	Dark-green leafy vegetables, liver, and fruits
Biotin	Aids in energy production	Egg yolks, liver, beans, and nuts
Pantothenic acid	Aids in energy production; aids in the manufacture of fatty acids; participates in a wide variety of other biochemical processes	Most foods

FIGURE A6.6 Vitamins. (Source: Reprinted with permission from *Eat for Life,* National Academy Press, Washington DC, 1992. Courtesy of the National Academy Press.)

Mineral	Functions	Food Sources
Calcium	The most abundant mineral in the body, 99 percent is in bones; is also important in muscle function	Dairy products, bones of sardines and canned calmon, dark-green leafy vegetables, and lime-processed tortillas
Chloride	Is a component of stomach acid; aids in maintaining fluid balance in cells	Table salt, eggs, meat, and milk
Chromium	Works with insulin to promote carbohydrate and fat metaqbolism	Liver and other organ meats, brewer's yeast, whole grains, and nuts
Copper	Aids in energy production; aids in absorption of iron from digestive tract; forms dark pigment in hair and skin	Liver, meat, whole grains, and nuts
Fluoride	Strengthens teeth and bones	Some natural waters, fluoridated water, and tea
Iodine	Is part of the thyroid hormones that regulate metabolism	Iodized table salt, ocean seafood, dairy products, and commercially made bread
Iron	Aids in energy production; helps to carry oxygen in the blood stream and muscles	Meat, poultry, fish, nuts, whole and enriched grain products, and green vegetables
Magnesium	Is necessary for nerve function, bone formation, and general metabolic processes	Grain products, vegetables, dairy products, fish, meat, and poultry
Manganese	Aids in regulation of carbohydrate metabolism and in general metabolic processes	Cereals and most other plant foods
Molybdenum	Aids in energy production	Meat, beans, and cereals
Phosphorus	Aids in bone formation, general metabolic processes, and energy production and storage	Dairy products, meat, poultry, fish, and grain products
Potassium	Is necessary to maintain fluid balance in cells, transmit nerve signals, and produce energy	Fruits and vegetables, nuts, grains, and seeds
Selenium	Protects cells against harmful reactions involving oxygen; aids in detoxifying toxic substances	Meat, ocean fish, and wheat
Sodium	Is necessary to maintain fluid balance in cells, transmit nerve signals, and relax muscles	Table salt and salt added to food during processing
Zinc	Is necessary for cell reproduction and tissue repair and growth	Oysters and other shellfish, meat, poultry, eggs, hard cheeses, milk, yogurt, beans, nuts, and whole-grain cereals

FIGURE A6.7 Minerals. (Source: Reprinted with permission from *Eat for Life,* National Academy Press, Washington DC, 1992. Courtesy of the National Academy Press.)

Index

A

B

E

F

G

H

I

J

K

L

M

N

Q

R

S

T

U

V

W

X

Z